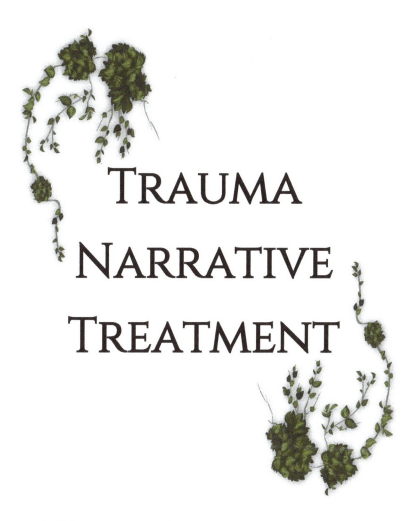

Trauma Narrative Treatment

A Trauma Recovery Model for Groups

2ND EDITION

W. David Lane, Ph.D.
Donna E. Lane, Ph.D.

©Copyright 2018 by W. David Lane and Donna E. Lane
All rights reserved

This manual is intended for use by the purchaser and may not be replicated, reprinted, distributed, or used for any other purpose without the expressed written consent of the authors of the model. All rights are reserved for this material, its printing, copying, use, and distribution.

ISBN: 978-1-7328112-1-8

Cover art by Lars Nissen

This model is intended for use with the story, Gold Stone, by David and Donna Lane.

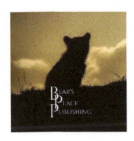

BEAR'S PLACE PUBLISHING
Snellville, GA

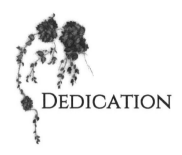DEDICATION

To the people of Haiti:
Romans 5:3-5
Romans 8:28

To Cody, who wrote his story of love and miracles

Table of Contents

Acknowledgements	5
Preface	7
Using the Model	9
Introduction	10
Understanding Trauma	14
What is Trauma?	14
What Happens During Trauma?	15
What are the Effects of Trauma?	16
What are the Results of Trauma?	25
How is Loss Related to Trauma?	33
The Trauma Narrative Model	35
How Does the Model Address Trauma?	35
What Does the Research Say?	38
What is Narrative?	39
How Does Creative Expression Help?	44
Why Groups?	47
Leader Skills	47
How Does This Model Work?	57
Lesson 1: Introduction and Overview	63
Lesson 2: Life Before the Trauma	67
Lesson 3: The Traumatic Event	71
Lesson 4: Life After the Trauma	77
Lesson 5: Defining Life from Now Forward	81
Lesson 6: Review and Evaluation	87
Bibliography	92
About the Authors	97
The Artists	99

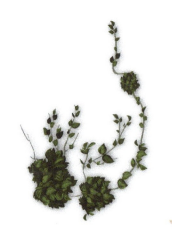

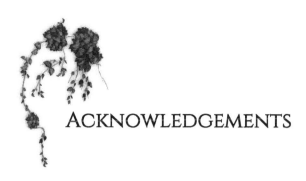

ACKNOWLEDGEMENTS

We are very grateful to all the people who have been involved in the writing, field testing, and research for the development of these materials. Chief among them, we are thankful for the openness and acceptance of the Haitian people, who were willing to bravely share their own stories with us, as they began the process of preparing to rise from the ashes of their losses. Their resilience is the most powerful symbol of writing a different story for the future that I can think of. It is our sincere hope that these materials continue to impact individuals with hope and healing, inspiring others to share and write their own endings to their stories.

Others who helped immensely:

Elizabeth Norris, Ralph Menard, Keith Myers, Stan Hoover, Sarah Amuka, Brittany Brown, and Auvronette Guilbeaux, Mercer University graduate students who helped immensely with the literature review and editing;

Bloodine Bobb-Semple and Rose Donatien, both Mercer students who traveled to Haiti as part of the training team to do the training workshops for the Haitian volunteers. Both of these wonderful bilingual ladies were Haitian Creole speakers and provided wonderful expertise and boundless energy for the project;

Olivier Clermont, a Haitian native and Mercer graduate student who made every trip to Haiti with me to act as translator and facilitator. This project would not have been possible without Olivier and the graciousness of his family who hosted us for each visit in Port au Prince and Jeremie;

Dr. Kenyon Knapp and Dr. Linda Foster, Mercer faculty members who participated in trips to Haiti and were instrumental in the workshop training sessions;

Dr. Charles Tardieu and the University of Jeremie Project, Jeremie, Haiti: Dr. Tardieu is former Minister of Education for Haiti and was instrumental in arranging meetings with various dignitaries and leaders who helped connect us to groups desiring training. Dr. Tardieu hosted a week-long training for 85 teachers in Jeremie, Haiti;

Dr. Joel Dorsinville and the Haitian Baptist Fellowship who carved out time in their annual Haitian Baptist Convention, got us on the agenda for training, and helped facilitate the training for 133 pastors at the Christian University of North Haiti in Cap Haitian, Haiti;

Dr. Rosalie Benjamin and Dr. Ginette Maguet of Institut de Developpement Personnel et Organisationnel (IDEO), Port au Prince, Haiti, who coordinated and hosted a week-long training for 21 community volunteers at the IDEO facility. Dr. Benjamin had been tasked by the Haitian Health Ministry to coordinate mental health relief efforts and provided valuable information and linkages to individuals and groups for training and intervention;

The Cooperative Baptist Fellowship, who provided funds and personnel support to carry out the work in Haiti. Special thanks to Dr. Daniel Vestal, Dr. Harry Rowland, and Dr. Reid Doster for their support, friendship, and encouragement;

Dr. Jim Jennings of Conscience International, who surprised me one day out of the blue with the idea for the Haiti work, provided funding for the travel and trainings, and who continues to solicit my input and involve me in projects in areas of need throughout the world; and to Mercer University, a teaching and service oriented university, the likes of which could only be matched, never exceeded.

Wilton Baptist Church, Wilton, CT, and Pastor Jason Coker, who hosted a community training in the use of these materials following the shootings at Sandy Hook Elementary School, and who allowed us to return at the anniversary of the shooting to follow up with the participants on the status of their community.

Marie Paddock, who took the materials to Rwanda to work with trauma survivors of the Rwandan genocide, and who provided anecdotal data showing the efficacy of the program.

We know we have left some people and agencies out. Please forgive us. It is our error alone. We hope you know that it goes without saying that we stand on the shoulders of giants.

David and Donna Lane

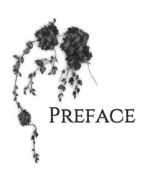

PREFACE

The genesis of this concept of a group treatment curriculum based on narrative came from the work we did in Haiti after the earthquake in 2010. I (David) was called in early spring, 2010, by Dr. Jim Jennings, CEO of Conscience International, an international, nongovernmental organization that, among other things, provides disaster relief and support in troubled areas around the world. Jim's group had moved immediately on January 10, 2010, in response to the devastating earthquake that left several hundred thousand dead and injured, and approximately four million people displaced. Jim and his volunteers were on the ground in Haiti for the better part of two months working round the clock with the injured and displaced. After the immediate survival needs had been addressed, Jim recognized the extreme need for psychological first aide and trauma care, so he called me.

As founding faculty member and (at the time) Coordinator of the graduate counseling programs at Mercer University, I have been privileged to train hundreds of counselors and to work extensively in the areas of trauma and Post Traumatic Stress Disorder. Jim wanted to put together a program for Haiti to train Haitians to assess and work with the traumatized population. Through the generous funding of the Cooperative Baptist Fellowship and Mercer University, I was able to travel to Haiti to assess the need and meet with key individuals to develop strategies for the most appropriate intervention methods.

In my meetings with Haitian leaders, pastors, and teachers, it quickly became apparent that Haiti has a story-telling culture, and it seemed most appropriate to use narrative based interventions. While still in Haiti I called my wife, Donna, and told her about my idea to develop a narrative group-oriented training program with a story as the central focal point of the program. We thought it would be ideal to use actual Haitian history as the story's backdrop. After some initial research on the history and culture of the region, we decided the story would be focused on the trauma to the Arawak culture from the Spaniards landing on Hispaniola. Using figures from Arawak history with whom the Haitian people still identify, along with some other common American and West African symbols to include other elements of the Haitian culture today, we decided on an approach for writing the central story. The next day I called Donna and she informed me the story was ready; that she had prayed about it the night before and had awakened with the entire story formulated in her mind. It had taken her about four hours to write down what she stated God had given to her as the whole story.

After I came home from that first Haiti trip, with the groups we were to train identified and a plan for the curriculum to train the volunteer trauma workers, Donna and I finalized the story, making it the centerpiece of trauma materials designed to address the issues of psychological first aid, trauma assessment, and group care for trauma victims. We wanted to ensure that it was "user friendly" because pastors, teachers, and community volunteers would not be trained therapists and would not have a counseling, psychology, or social sciences background. And so, the essence of this curriculum was born.

In three ensuing trips, we were able to train multiple groups of pastors, teachers, and community workers, and assess the efficacy of the materials by testing the participants in the program for changes in trauma-related symptomatology after completion. The story resonated with the Haitian people with whom we were working and is still being used today by the over 230 volunteers that we trained.

Since then, the Cooperative Baptist Fellowship has funded work in Newtown, CT, using the materials to train pastors and community workers to respond following the Sandy Hook shootings, and as a follow-up at the first anniversary of the shootings.

The story and materials have been used by mission groups in such locations as Rwanda, Cambodia, Malaysia, Jordan, Dominican Republic, Costa Rica, Vietnam, New Zealand, and China, the Middle East, and in multiple locations across the United States.

Using the Model

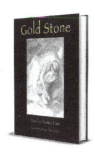

This model is intended for use with the story, Gold Stone (2014), by David and Donna Lane, available from Amazon, Barnes and Noble, and Regeneration Writers Press.

This model is intended for use with small groups but may be used with individuals as well. The goal of the model is to intervene following a traumatic experience toward preventing the development of severe mental health disorders as a consequence of the trauma. It may be adapted for use by mental health professionals to address individuals who have developed mental health disorders as a result of their trauma, but that use requires clinical training and expertise in dealing with these complex issues. Individuals suffering from complex trauma, dissociative disorders, suicidal ideation, or other mental health disorders that make group participation difficult or impossible should be referred to a mental health professional for a more appropriate level of mental health care.

To the leader: Please read the *Understanding Trauma* and *The Trauma Narrative Model* sections of this manual carefully, so you can understand how trauma affects and changes us and what the participants are experiencing, before you begin leading the group. An understanding of these processes is essential to responding appropriately to the group members' needs.

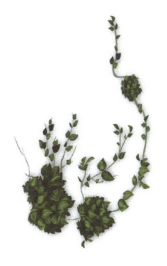

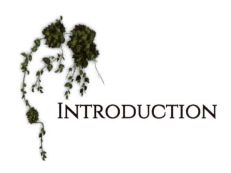

Introduction

What is your story?

April-July, 1994, Rwandan genocide; September 11. 2001, New York, Washington, and Pennsylvania, terrorist attack; March 11, 2004, Madrid train bombings; December 26, 2004, India earthquake and Thailand tsunami; August 29, 2005, Louisiana and Mississippi, US, Hurricane Katrina; May 12, 2008, China earthquake; January 12, 2010, Haitian earthquake; February 22, 2011, New Zealand earthquake; March 15, 2011 through today, Syrian refugee crisis; April 13. 2013, Boston Marathon bombings, Boston, Massachusetts; January 3-7, Nigeria, Baga Massacre; January 2015 through today, Myanmar Rohingya refugee crisis; April 25, 2015, Nepal earthquake; September 7, 2017, Mexican earthquake; August 2018, California wildfires. This list is a sampling of the variety of traumatic experiences without number that hundreds of thousands have experienced, just in the last twenty-five years.

Not limited to terror attacks or natural disasters, trauma for individuals takes many forms: witnessing or experiencing violent crimes; rape and/or sexual abuse; physical abuse and domestic violence; the devastation of war and postwar displacement; loss of a loved one; accidents; protracted illness; any circumstance that puts life and limb at risk. These examples of trauma affect almost everyone at some point in their lives.

Each day, countless individuals wake up in the morning and the sun is shining, and they feel loved. However, just a short time later, nothing is the same. What do you do when everything you have ever known, everyone you have ever loved, your life as you know it is suddenly changed – wiped away, evaporated, disappeared? Do you quit? Do you run away? Do you decide you want to just die and not face it anymore? Do you even want to go on?

Prior to the occurrence of a traumatic event or events, certain basic assumptions guide your life: assumptions like self-determination, basic safety and security, environmental stability, the coming of tomorrow, the presence of the people you love. Then trauma strikes. Suddenly, you are vulnerable, and your world is no longer safe and secure. Furthermore, you can't make sense of what is left in the aftermath.

There are many reactions you might have. Initially, you may feel shock, terror, or a sense that what happened is unreal or surreal. You may feel numb, as if you have left your body, or you may feel disconnected from or unaware of everything around you. Memories might flash before your eyes in horrifying fragments, or you may not even remember all the details (or any of the details) of what just happened. The images of the trauma might replay over and over again, disrupting thought and sleep. New experiences following the trauma may continue to feel depersonalized, meaning they are not connected to you, as if you are watching a movie or the experiences are happening to someone else, and your ability to integrate those new experiences into your life story may be compromised. You may find yourself replaying the trauma in your interactions with others through your assumptions and beliefs. Confronted with the reality of inescapable shock, your mental and bodily systems may begin to break down (Meichenbaum, 2017; Van Der Kolk, 2014).

Many factors impact how you react to a traumatic event: your age (younger persons often react more significantly than older persons); what or who produces the trauma (if a loved one is the agent of traumatic experience, the impact is much more severe); the amount of preparation time you had prior to the event (for example, a hurricane may have several days' notice, while an earthquake has little or no forewarning); the amount of damage done to you (physically, emotionally, and spiritually) or to your property; the amount of death and devastation you witness; the degree of responsibility you feel for causing or not preventing the event; your previous experiences of adversity or trauma; the level of support you have available to you before, during, and after the trauma; your attachment style. These are just some of the factors that can impact your reactions to a major traumatic event.

The results of trauma are manifold, including loss of a sense of self; disrupted or fragmented memory; numbing of your depth of feeling, with the exception of rage or shame when a memory of the trauma is triggered; reorganization of perception, where the trauma is superimposed on everything around you; loss of imagination and mental flexibility, which impacts coping; immobilization or agitation due to increased secretion of stress hormones, resulting in hyper-reactivity to all stimuli; loss of agency, resulting in mental paralysis and interruption in decision-making; and compromised ability to function socially (Van Der Kolk, 2014).

If trauma occurred earlier in life, it does not mean the impact of the trauma is lessened. In fact, early childhood experiences of trauma are often more devastating, because the child has fewer resources with which to cope, and the consequences extend into adulthood. Whether the trauma occurred in the distant past or more recently, the individual experiences the trauma as if it is happening in their present, due to the different way the traumatic memories are stored and accessed in the brain.

Almost everyone, by the time they reach adulthood, has experienced some form of trauma in their lives. We developed this model using the most current research on trauma recovery, combining the most effective methods to maximize effectiveness and bring healing. What is your story of trauma? How have your experiences impacted you? Do you relate to any of these reactions and results listed? This model is designed to address and help ameliorate the responses to trauma that are normal responses to horrible circumstances but are disruptive to healthy functioning and successful daily living. Through this process, you can come to understand that trauma does not define you or determine the course of your life.

The six-session model uses techniques demonstrated through research to be effective in addressing trauma, using a story entitled *Gold Stone*, which can be easily shared and relates directly to individuals who have experienced trauma. The story addresses the major elements that may be experienced as a result of trauma, including death, profound loss of relationship, life-altering environmental changes, feelings of guilt and self-blame, rage, powerlessness, depersonalization and derealization, loss of a sense of self, and spiritual questioning.

Using the story as a reference point, participants in small groups share their own personal stories leading up to the trauma. Following along with the main character of the story, participants then share their trauma experiences. Finally, participants begin the process of finding meaning in their experiences, reconnecting with their sense of self to reestablish wholeness, and choosing how their story will proceed following the trauma.

If the curriculum is being used in response to a natural disaster or terrorist attack, many care providers can be trained in the model by small numbers of professionals, promoting a strong sense of "communities helping themselves" while creating a resource multiplying effect for individuals who have experienced disaster-related trauma. Using community resources allows intervention to take place immediately, and the six-session structure of the model allows the intervention to be brief, addressing the needs specific to a region or area recovering from a disaster, with the goals of preventing the development of long term trauma-related pathology and promoting healing.

Let's begin by understanding more about what constitutes trauma and the consequences in the lives of individuals who go through traumatic experiences.

Trauma is...

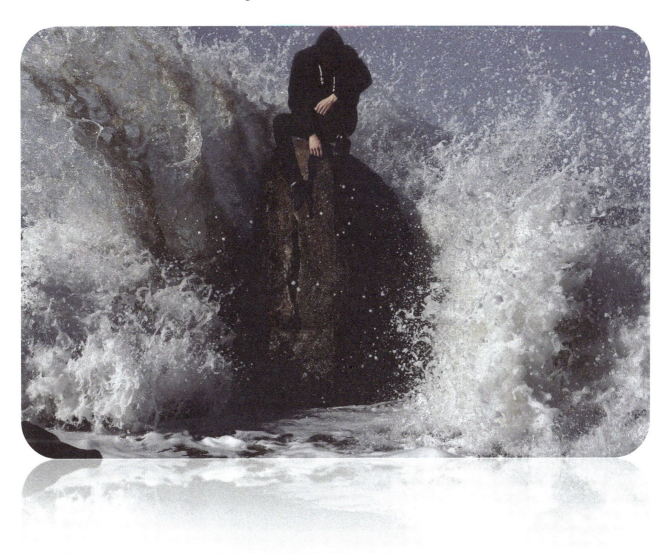

like waves crashing
against the
sand and rocks
on the shore

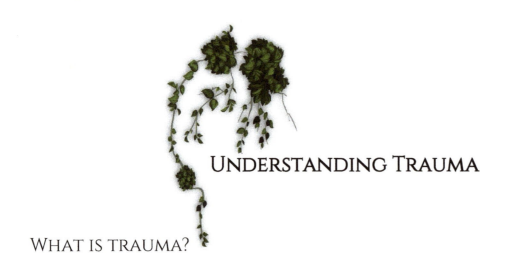

Understanding Trauma

What is trauma?

Trauma is an emotional response to a severely distressing event or series of events that overwhelms an individual's ability and capacity to cope. Anything that interrupts the integration of the emotions involved in an experience would be considered traumatic.

Trauma can occur in many forms; however, three main types of trauma are recognized, with each one bearing different consequences. The first type of trauma is a dramatic event or experience which shocks the system but at some point, comes to an end. The second type is an ongoing, continually distressing series of events or experiences from which there is no foreseeable relief. The third type of trauma is vicarious or secondary trauma, which occurs from being close to or in relationship with someone who is going through or has gone through trauma.

The first type of trauma is like a ball-peen hammer against a sheet of glass, the glass representing the internal structure of the personality. Depending on a variety of factors (the thickness of the glass, the weight of the hammer, the force of the swing, the number of previous hits), the glass can be left with a single ding, or spider-web cracks; larger fragmenting cracks, with broken out pieces; or, completely shattered in pieces on the ground, with nothing left in the frame but a huge hole.

The second type of trauma is more like waves against the sand and rocks on the shore. At first, you don't see much happening, but the constant flow of water and recurrent crashing of the waves undermines the foundation of the land. It erodes the sand, wears down the resistance, and cuts into the rock. The constant pressure begins to leave deep gullies where the flow of water begins to collect, and soon the gulley turns into a canyon. Eventually, the sand is washed away, the dune collapses, and the foundation is swept away in the waves.

Secondary trauma is like standing some distance from the center of a bomb blast but still experiencing a shock wave after the blast occurs. The immediate impact of the trauma itself is not experienced, but the aftereffects and consequences of the trauma are, and it can impact the individual and drain life energy in a way similar to experiencing the trauma. Vicarious or secondary trauma can impact loved ones living in the home with the traumatized person, close friends and extended family, and professionals working with the trauma survivor in a caregiver role.

For all three forms of trauma, certain consequences and responses are consistently present. Let's go over what causes these responses.

What happens during trauma?

When a frightening or distressing event happens, adrenaline is pumped in increasing amounts into the system. This extra adrenaline is related to the fight/flight/freeze response that is intended for survival, and it helps, but only up to the point when the system is overwhelmed. When the body system becomes inundated with the sensory data coming in, the integrated functioning of the system begins to break down. The frontal lobe, the part of the brain involved in reason and cognition, shuts down (Lacona & Johnson, 2018).

When cognitive processing shuts down, the individual is no longer able to put feelings into words, making it difficult for them to make sense of the traumatic experience. They lose their sense of location and time. The raw data is no longer processed properly, so their memory of the traumatic event cannot be stored in their long-term memory as other memories are. Instead, the traumatic experience is stored in a different part of the brain as flashes of fragmented sensory and emotional traces (Van der Kolk, 2014).

As a result, traumatic memories are not stored as logical, coherent narratives and are not integrated into the individual's story. Any frame of reference for the experience is lost, which creates a loss of perspective. Our memories are typically compared against the overarching story of our lives, providing a frame of reference for the new experience within the context of our whole story. However, an individual going through trauma loses all frame of reference. The individual has no ability to say, "that was then, this is now" (Meichenbaum, 2017). Because of this process, individuals experience the trauma as a present, here-and-now reality, even if the trauma happened many years ago.

When the traumatic memories are triggered, which can happen through random, transient events, such as smelling a particular smell associated with the trauma, sounds or tastes associated with the trauma, visual cues, physical stimuli, or a sudden movement that startles them, the individual is flooded with the whole sensory experience of the trauma, and they react as if the trauma is occurring in real time, because for their brain, it is (Lacona & Johnson, 2018). Just like happens during the original trauma, the frontal lobe shuts down and the ability to process the trauma logically and place it in some perspective is lost.

In addition, the brain becomes accustomed to the continuous flow of adrenaline. The body repeatedly reignites the stress hormones' release, resulting in the body itself replaying the trauma, even when the specific trauma memory is not triggered. The wear and tear on the body is significant (Lacona & Johnson, 2018).

The individual is haunted by shadows of bodily sensations and fragments of experience they cannot put into language (Crawford, 2010). Their experience of their lives becomes divided between body and mind, and this dissociation in and of itself is disconcerting. The individual begins to feel they must either shut down completely to deal with the overwhelming sensations, or they live in a state of hyperarousal, responding out of proportion to everything going on around them.

Memories are the stories of ourselves. Stories give shape to our lives, and even give substance to our very selves (Scheib, 2016). Our stories serve a specific purpose, helping us make sense of our experiences, placing us in and connecting us to reality, giving meaning to our lives, and helping us identify who we are. However, traumatic memories, those fragments or flashes of sensory experience without the rational component of our brains coming to bear, do not serve this purpose (Van der Kolk, 2014). They become rigid and inflexible. They prevent us from connecting to ourselves or others. They mire us in the distressing experience, which we relive over and over again each time the traumatic memory is triggered, with no resolution, no meaning, and no ability to integrate the memory into our overall story. You can see how the consequences of trauma could be severe.

WHAT ARE THE EFFECTS OF TRAUMA?

Trauma can have a profound, even devastating impact on an individual. Often, the responses traumatized individuals exhibit are pathologized (Johnson, 2018). They are viewed as needing "treatment" and are identified as "disturbed." The truth is, the responses we list below to trauma are "normal" responses given the extreme nature of their situation. Pathologizing the person or seeing the person as a problem hinders the successful integration of the trauma memories into their overall life story (Pack, 2008). We must recognize these responses are normal for their experience and are based on real physiological and emotional reactions in the body and mind of the individual to a traumatic event.

If we normalize the response to trauma, we increase the likelihood the individual will be open to explore their experiences, which in turn increases the opportunity for the individual to give language to their trauma. If they can give language to their trauma, they can begin the process of including the traumatic experience into their overall life story. The brain systems that handle self-awareness can begin to alter the bodily responses that feel so out of control and out of context. Finally, the individual can begin to rediscover their identity through giving language to their inner reality (Hutto, et al., 2017).

Helping individuals who have gone through trauma understand their responses are normal, and they are not alone in experiencing these responses, can help open the doors to the process of healing. Below we have listed some of the "normal," expected responses to trauma.

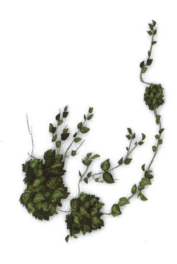

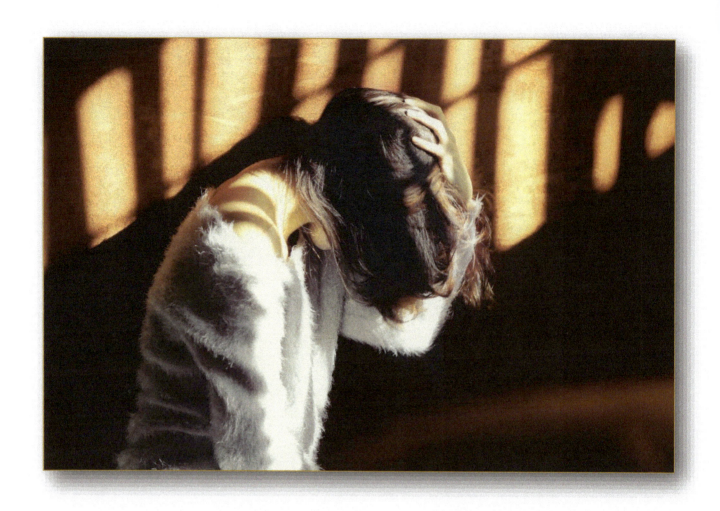

Responses to trauma are normal responses to abnormal circumstances

LOSS OF BODY AWARENESS

During and after traumatic experiencing, systems for physical regulation, such as respiration, the circulatory system, digestion, hormone regulation, and the immune system, become overwhelmed by the perceived sense of threat. The body's responses become "stuck" in shock-mode. The individual exists in a perpetual state of agitation or complete shut-down, living in the extremes of experience. Neural responses are slowed, and neural activity is delayed in the brain regions necessary for cognitive processing (Hall, et al, 2018). Trauma, particularly early trauma, alters neural pathways in the brain, changes neurological structure and function, and leads to somatic problems (Thomason, et al., 2017).

Think about what happens when someone's body goes into a state of shock. The blood flow leaves the extremities and centers on vital systems only. The frontal lobe of the brain shuts down, leaving the more primitive parts of the brain to run things. The individual begins to feel disconnected from their own body and mind, and when they lose their sense of their body, they lose their sense of themselves.

LOSS OF SELF

One of the initial effects of trauma is a loss of sensory self-awareness. The areas of the brain that work together to create a sense of self, which typically activate when the brain is in "rest" mode, cannot activate because the brain remains constantly activated toward survival of the threat (Van Der Kolk, 2014). Knowing what we feel leads to knowing why we feel it which leads to mobilization of resources to manage and respond to those feelings. None of these normal responses occur in the presence of extreme disconnection from the self. Because disconnection from self continues well after the traumatic event is over, these responses also continue to occur. As a result, the individual loses their sense of purpose and direction, the feeling of being alive, and the sense of who they are. They no longer feel in charge of their own life.

LOSS OF AGENCY

Agency is the feeling of overseeing one's own life. When trauma, such as natural disasters like an earthquake, hurricane, or fire, or man-made trauma like sexual abuse, rape, or other acts of violence, sweeps into their lives, their sense of personal authority is swept away with it. Something or someone external to their ability to choose overpowers them, leaving them feeling vulnerable, out of control, and powerless. Because they have no choice about experiencing the traumatic event, their feelings tell them they have no choice at all. Their sense of basic safety and security is lost, as is their belief they can self-determine.

Often, this personal paralysis extends into all decision-making, and trauma survivors become chameleons who acquiesce to the desires of those around them instead of choosing based on their own desires. It doesn't take long for the individual to lose sight of their own desires completely, which leads to a disconnection from all feeling.

Numbing

The loss of emotional connectivity may be very confusing. At times, individuals who have experienced trauma may wonder why they cannot feel the depth of love they once felt, or the excitement and joy they expect to feel during a special event; instead, a sudden onset of deep shame or a sense of rage that does not appear connected to anything in their present arises seemingly from nowhere. Often, these individuals are not aware of the triggers that stir up the sensations of being in the middle of the traumatic event. It can be something as innocuous as a smell that reminds them of the day of the trauma or an association with an object that pulls a memory fragment back to the surface. The numbing of emotions may be the response to the intrusion of those memory fragments (Crawford, 2010). The rational is disconnected from the emotional, so the individual can no longer make sense of what they are experiencing. Their emotions, or lack thereof, become a jumble of disconnected messages and sensations that they cannot link as a part of their story.

Superimposition of Trauma

The way a trauma memory is stored and where it is stored in the brain is different from regular memories. Trauma memory has no orientation in time and place. When a stimulus triggers the trauma memory, the individual's experience of the original trauma superimposes over their current circumstances. Intrusive images and sensations make it seem to the traumatized individual that the trauma is happening in the present (Leahy, 2009). They are unable to distinguish the where and when of the trauma or place it in any context, and they may have great difficulty deciphering what is going on around them.

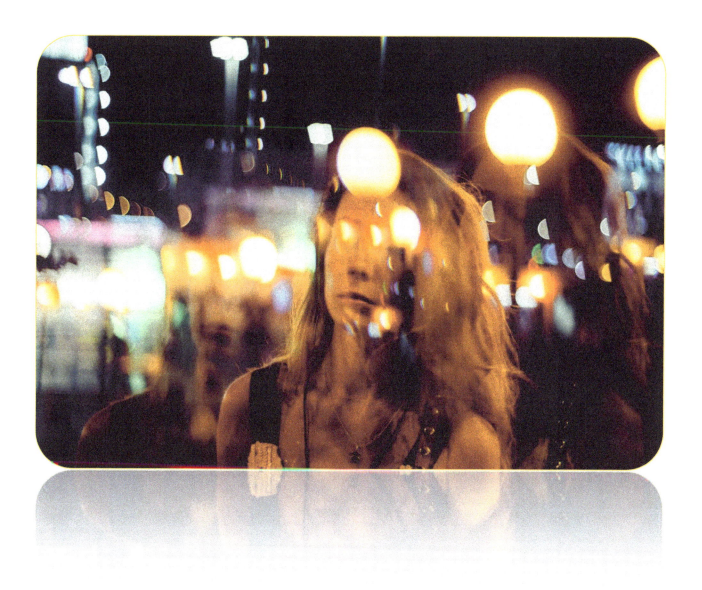

Intrusive images and sensations make it seem that the trauma is happening in the present.

Any stranger walking by on the street may be perceived as a threat. A balloon popping or a large truck rumbling by on the road may be heard as a bomb exploding or the beginning of another earthquake. Their spouse walking up behind them may be responded to as someone coming to kill or hurt them. The smell of supper burning on the stove may cause panic as if the house is burning down around them. Someone touching their arm or tapping them on the shoulder may be perceived as the warning signal for impending abuse. As a result, everywhere they turn is a potential perceived threat to their survival, and the threat is unrelenting. Their body and mind believe they must remain on alert at all times to deal with the impending danger. The physical and emotional consequences of remaining on high alert are numerous.

Agitation or Immobilization

The levels of stress hormones in individuals who have gone through trauma, even well after the experience itself is over, is much higher than normal (Van Der Kolk, 2014). The presence of these hormones leaves them hyperreactive, sending a neurological and biochemical signal throughout the body that keeps them feeling agitated or immobilized, like a bunny cornered in a cave with a wolf at the entrance. They may find themselves in a cyclical response of hyperarousal followed by hypoarousal, where they shut down to deal with the overwhelming affective and bodily sensations they are experiencing (Crawford, 2010). The fight/flight/freeze response is always active. The individual may erupt unexpectedly over a small, insignificant slight, or they may freeze at the smallest confrontation or disagreement. Either way, their response is out of proportion to the current situation; instead, it is a response appropriate to threat of death. These responses impact the individual in every way, including physically, emotionally, mentally, and socially.

Physiological responses

The constant stress in the body from the continuous presence of stress hormones, the cycle of hyperarousal, and the out-of-proportion responses can result in a myriad of physiological consequences, such as headaches, blood pressure issues, heart problems, chronic fatigue, diabetes, digestive problems, and autoimmune disorders. When emotional responses are shut down, the body tends to somaticize feelings, meaning the feelings are expressed physically through pain and illness.

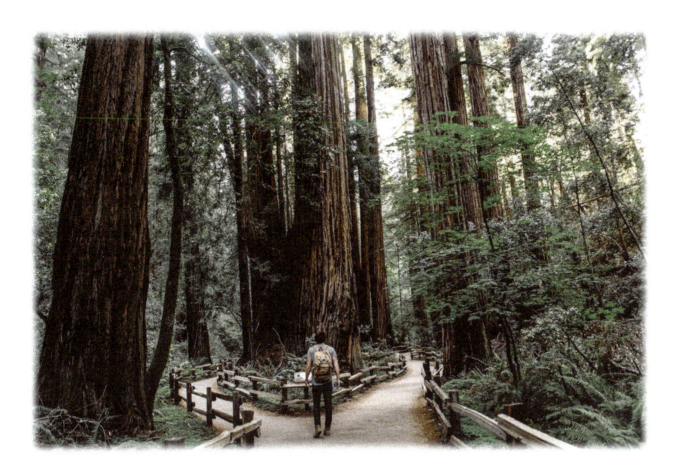

The brain is rigidly stuck repeating the same destructive choices, unable to imagine alternatives

Rigidity

Remaining on high alert produces mental rigidity, which results in a loss of imagination and creativity (Van der Kolk, 2014). The ability to imagine is what makes problem solving possible. Without imagination, the brain is stuck with repeating strategies that have been tried before. The traumatized individual may find themselves repeating the same unsuccessful behaviors, even though they are consciously aware those responses did not work in the past, simply because they cannot think of anything else to try. Their brain gets stuck in "ruts" like car tracks on old dirt roads that are dug out by repetitive driving over the same ground day after day. Flexibility, which is a sign of mental health, is lost, and coping skills are limited. They may even feel compelled to revisit experiences that remind them of the trauma, although it may be terrifying to do so, because their brain is saying it must drive in the "ruts" on the road.

At the same time, the brain remains attached to the trauma, repetitively recreating the traumatic experience, and is unable to successfully integrate the trauma with new experiences or into their life story, resulting in being rigidly stuck in the developmental stage where the trauma occurred. A slow and steady decline in the ability to function in the here-and-now of life is the result.

Impaired Social Functioning

Human beings are designed to be social creatures. As a result, social connectivity is necessary for healthy functioning and fulfillment. The inability to function adequately in the social context is at the root of a lot of human suffering, whether the dysfunction is the result of difficulty in creating healthy relationships or the result of problems with self-regulation around others. Because trauma leaves the individual feeling disconnected from themselves, it also produces a feeling of being disconnected from others. As a result, reciprocity, which is the sense of being seen and heard and known by the people around you, is lost (Van Der Kolk, 2014). Relationships are no longer satisfying and potential support networks are lost. If they cannot connect, they cannot function in a social context.

Changes in Memory

Emotionally charged events are generally better retained in long term memory and are more readily accessible for recall; however, when the event reaches the level of trauma, memory retention and integration changes. The brain's system for storing memory is overwhelmed in the presence of horror and terror, the frontal lobe of the brain shuts down, the primitive brain is left activated, feelings can no longer be put into words, the orientation to location and time is lost, information coming in through the senses is interrupted, and proper integration and storage of that information is prevented (Van Der Kolk, 2014).

As a result, the traumatic experiences are no longer stored as a narrative that is logical, ordered, and understandable; instead, the memories are stored as fragments of sensation and emotion, with little or no story line. Memories are like stories, with a beginning, a middle, and an end. They are oriented in time and space, with a frame of reference. However, traumatic memories have no connection to the overarching story of the individual's life. Thus, they have no perspective to balance the experience or context within which to understand the experience and give it meaning.

WHAT ARE THE RESULTS OF TRAUMA?

Dissociation, meaning internal disconnection, or the separation of mental processes that are normally related or connected, is the primary result of trauma. Imagine the individual's body as a home. For most people, life is lived in the main areas, with occasional visits to private spaces for reflection and self-awareness, but all the areas of the home are connected and integrated. The individual is able to move freely and easily from space to space, without losing their connection to the rest of the home. However, the traumatized individual's inner "home" is no longer safe or secure. Their brain constructs a long, dark corridor, a passageway into a closed-off, isolated room from which the individual can observe life, but is not connected to it. Life goes on in the main part of the house while the individual watches from a "safe" and unreachable distance. A hologram of themselves may be projected into the main area to give others the impression that they are present and participating, but the individual is emotionally shut down and unavailable. They can no longer access or move freely through the rest of their home.

Trauma is an external event that rips apart their lives. The emotional result of trauma is a feeling that everything has been torn apart or lost, including their sense of who they are. As discussed, there is a pattern to this tearing: memories of the trauma become disconnected, fragmented images and sensations rather than a fluid story with a beginning, a middle, and an ending; the difference between the present and the past is lost to them, as the trauma invades the present and dictates their responses; they lose their ability to self-regulate and, in a constant state of arousal, they struggle with creating satisfying relationships and functioning in the here-and-now; their sense of self and of being in charge of their own lives is lost to them; not knowing what they feel or why they feel it leads to an inability to mobilize resources to manage life; triggers that remind them of the trauma result in involuntary and repetitive response patterns that recreate the trauma experience but are not connected or appropriate to the present circumstances, leaving them feeling out of control and out of sync with life; ultimately, they feel like an observer of life rather than someone present in it. This is the essence of dissociation. As Langer (1991) describes it, "Life goes on, but in two temporal directions at once, the future unable to escape the grip of a memory laden with grief."

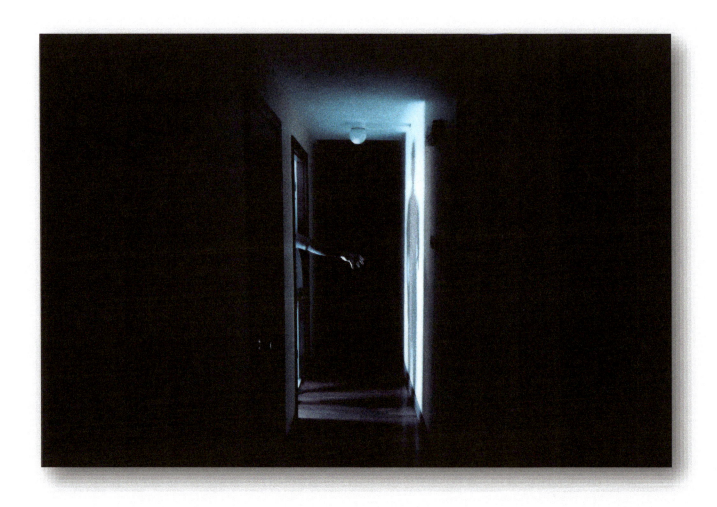

The brain constructs a dark passageway into an isolated room from which they observe life, but are not connected to it

Their experience of the trauma remains separated from their life story, as if it happened to someone else, and disconnected from what they would otherwise experience as a secure and predictable present, dividing their mind in such a way that nothing can seem secure and predictable. The trauma itself is unimaginable and unbearable, while day-to-day life goes on. It is as if they are living two lives: the daily experience of the trauma and the daily experiences of working and eating and sleeping and trying to relate in the present. Because they are unable to create meaning from the trauma by integrating it into their life story, the disconnected part of themselves is frozen in time and place.

The ongoing consequences of traumatic experience include feeling heaviness in the chest with difficulty breathing at times, tightening in the throat and holding tension in other areas of the body, remaining on constant alert, experiencing nightmares and flashbacks, disconnecting from self and others, feeling out of control, and staying in a kind of mental "fog" and emotional numbness that makes processing current experiences difficult (Van der Kolk, 2014).

In addition, their beliefs about themselves are altered based on the trauma. Self-loathing and shame are common beliefs, often because of the "freeze" aspect of the fight/flight/freeze response. Even though this response is involuntary, traumatized individuals often feel to blame, believing they "should" have done something to prevent the event. Along with shame beliefs, beliefs that they don't matter, are unimportant, have no purpose, or deserve what they got, are often present. If loved ones or others died during the trauma, feelings of guilt for surviving is a common result.

At the time of the trauma, these responses are not only a normal reaction to trauma but also a necessary response for the individual to continue to survive. Survival is always the first order of business; yet, these very survival responses begin to work against them, keeping them trapped in their pain. This can also perpetuate the need for the survival responses, creating a self-reinforcing cycle. The cycle of trauma becomes:

> "I need these (feelings/responses/thoughts/behaviors) to survive but these (feelings/responses/thoughts/behaviors) create more unpleasant (feelings/responses/thoughts/behaviors) that make me fear for my survival which creates more of these (feelings/responses/thoughts/behaviors) which makes me believe I need more of these (feelings/responses/thoughts) to survive."

Then the emotional trap is complete.

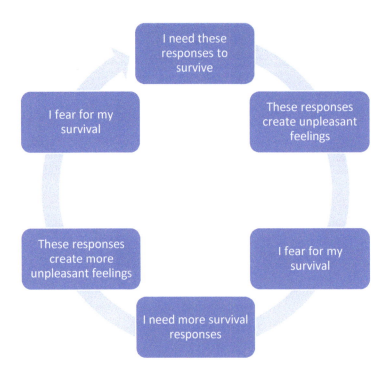

The individual feels fearful or hopeless or overwhelmed or insecure, and more survival response is required. Paradoxically, the harder they try to get over the trauma or deal with it by trying to bury it or change the unpleasant feelings, responses, and thoughts, the more those feelings, responses, and thoughts are reinforced. This pattern puts an enormous stress on the body and mind. Physical problems, such as autoimmune disorders, heart and blood pressure problems, digestive problems, and chronic fatigue, are often the result. The mind is also overwhelmed, and often shuts down rather than attempting to face the unfathomable. Physical actions create a context for mental processing, but trauma prohibits the appropriate physiological response and successful integration of experiences. The traumatized individual is haunted by bodily sensations and memory fragments that cannot be verbalized, and the body and mind are split as a result (Crawford, 2010).

Symptoms resulting from trauma can include re-experiencing the trauma in the form of nightmares, intrusive thoughts or memories, and flashbacks; disrupted sleep, irritability, exaggerated startled response, and hypervigilance; avoidance of places associated with the trauma, talking about the trauma, or associating with people connected to the trauma; constriction of emotion, shutting down, and suppression and repression. (Crawford, 2010). Their experience feels as if the past is invading the present or is still happening in the present.

SURVIVAL RESPONSES

Survival responses fall into four general categories:

1. <u>Feeling responsible for the traumatic event</u>

    This results from a feeling of having lost all sense of personal power and serves to help the trauma survivor feel a sense of power over the event. Frequently they feel guilt and shame associated with the event. They spend much of their time reviewing the events and trying to anticipate, prepare for, and prevent future trauma.

2. <u>Denial or loss of recollection that the event occurred</u>

    This serves to protect the traumatized individual from dealing with the horrific reality of the event. They may experience a total loss of memory, or they may forget significant details of the event. This may last for days, months, or even years. They most likely will recall the trauma at some point, and the memory may be triggered by a random event which may seem unrelated to the event itself. A milder form of denial is a minimization of the severity of the trauma which aids them in continuing to ignore the emotional pain and the torn identity.

3. <u>Harming self or others</u>

    This group of survival responses is much less socially acceptable and much more harmful. It serves the purpose of taking the focus off the internal pain and placing it on external objects or people. They want the pain to end, but they do not know how to make it stop. Self-injurious behaviors, such as cutting, substance abuse, eating disorders, and other types of self-harm may be attempts to make the pain stop or to feel something. Frequently, suicide is not intended to end the *life* but to end the *pain*. They respond to confrontation as an invitation to fight, which seems to bring some relief. Because of the nature of this type of response, it has the potential for permanent damage to self and others.

4. <u>Helping self and others</u>

    This form of survival response has no stigma attached and may not show any outward sign that they are actually attempting to cover internal pain and loss. Instead, most of these responses are applauded and strongly reinforced. They may focus on others' problems so much that they do not seem to have time to deal with their own pain.

The problem with these survival responses is that they serve two opposing purposes. They seem to provide some measure of relief while at the same time reinforcing the problem. Until these patterns become painful or do not work anymore, the traumatized individual will be likely to continue them on an unconscious level. This becomes even more problematic when they have experienced multiple traumas, or if their initial trauma occurred at a very young age (Thomson & Jaque, 2017).

WHY RESPONSES BECOME PROBLEMATIC

No one knows why some people seem to handle trauma better than others. Why do some people seem to manage, and some people seem to develop severe problems as a result of trauma? Research has demonstrated that someone with a secure attachment in earliest childhood is better equipped to cope with traumatic experiences, while those with insecure or disorganized attachments are more likely to develop dissociation and PTSD (Marshall & Frazier, 2018; Plokar, et al., 2018).

In addition, if the individual has a strong sense of self and what is known as an internal locus of control (which means they believe they are in charge of their own lives and events in their lives are primarily the results of their own actions) prior to the traumatic event, they are likely to handle the trauma better than someone who does not know who they are or someone who believes life happens to them instead of believing they are in charge of their life and actions prior to the trauma. These factors also explain, to some extent, why the age the first trauma is experienced directly impacts how devastating the trauma event will be, with earlier experiences having more destructive impact (Thomason & Marusak, 2017). Young children have not developed a strong sense of self and generally still see others (such as parents) or circumstances as in charge of their lives.

Finally, if individuals have a strong social network of support, and a supportive environment providing a feeling of safety, their chances of managing the trauma successfully are much higher than if they are isolated or their social network or community is unsupportive or abusive. Traumatized individuals need to feel seen and heard by those around them, recognized for who they are and not viewed as defined by their trauma, and allowed to function as a member of the social group to feel safe to share and heal.

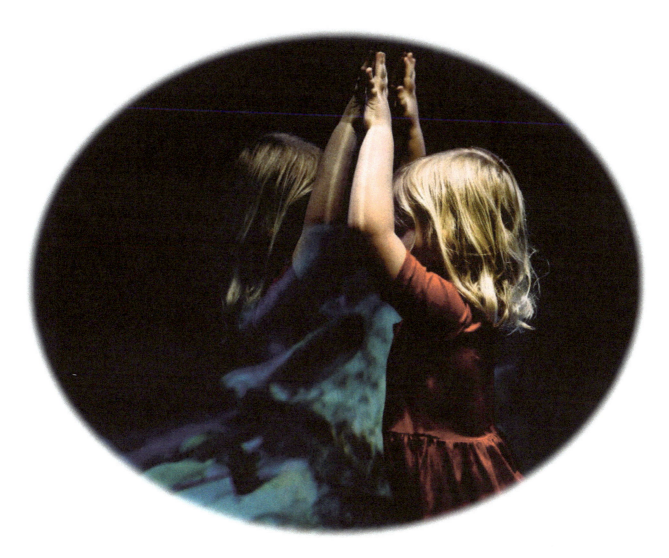

Children with secure attachments and a developing sense of self are better equipped to handle trauma

All the responses to trauma we have discussed are initially normal survival responses, and most people never develop extraordinary problems. However, most people *do* struggle to cope after trauma and may need some help overcoming their normal responses and difficulties of adjustment associated with traumatic experiencing. This program presents the kind of assistance that addresses those needs. Occasionally, however, responses to trauma can become pathological and develop into psychological disorders that need to be recognized, and the affected people need to be referred to a physician, psychologist, or counselor for further assistance.

Dealing with Trauma

Ordinary memory is basically a story we tell about our lives for a purpose (Van der Kolk, 2014). Our memories are flexible, even changing with retelling, creating a narrative that describes what we have experienced in the context of our whole story. However, traumatic memory is not flexible, not sequential, and serves no purpose, because it is stored as fragments of physical sensations and images, disconnected from language, so these memories cannot become part of their overarching story. The effects of trauma are ameliorated when the story can be put into words and shared in an environment of personal safety, so that the memory can be integrated with the emotion, given meaning, included in their overarching life story, and viewed as a past event instead of a present reality (Pack, 2008; Crawford, 2010; Van der Kolk, 2014).

Simply talking about the trauma is insufficient to deal with the trauma. If described from the disconnected view of someone relaying someone else's story, the memory will not be integrated into their life narrative, and they remain an observer rather than a participant in life. Their embodied experiences remain disconnected from their cognitive reality, and their physical and emotional selves remain dissociated (Carless & Douglas, 2016). If telling the traumatic event is not connected to the emotion from the event, the inner division described earlier remains intact, leaving them at war with themselves internally (Van der Kolk, 2014). Finally, the rational brain can make sense of emotion, but cannot alter the emotion; in other words, understanding why we feel does not change how we feel (Van der Kolk, 2014).

In order to give meaning to the trauma experience, the traumatized individual will need to connect to all aspects of the event, but only in the context of safety and support, having learned the ability to remain connected to mind and body and to have the voice and language to describe the experience with a beginning, a middle, and an ending (Pack, 2008). The trauma story must be integrated into their larger story, taken beyond memory fragments, sensations, and images into a narrative.

How is loss related to trauma?

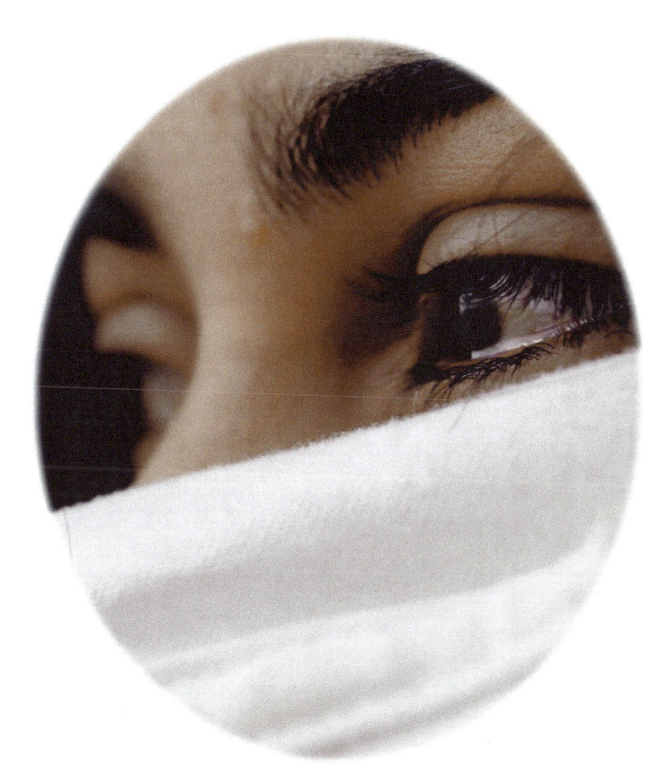

The grieving individual begins to collapse in on themselves, as if their very being is falling into that black hole of emptiness.

Loss is a type of trauma and can also be a compounding element in another traumatic experience, such as when the death of a loved one accompanies a traumatic event like an accident or natural disaster. Grief is the emotional experience resulting from loss. Many of the descriptors and consequences of trauma we have outlined are applicable to the experience of grief. For example, most individuals, when they experience a loss, feel an initial state of shock, where they struggle with processing the emotions they are feeling and with integrating those emotions and thoughts into their here-and-now experience. Many grieving individuals have difficulty accepting the loss as real and continue to "catch" themselves thinking of calling their loved one or expecting them to walk through the door. Events, holidays, anniversaries, birthdays, and familiar experiences can trigger deep emotional responses and pain for many years after the loss occurred.

The science of physics has demonstrated when two particles interact with one another in a vacuum and are later separated into two different containers, stimulating one particle produces an activation response in the other particle. In much the same way, when two individuals interact and form a relationship, an exchange of energy occurs between the two individuals. This attachment continues even when the two individuals are separated from one another by distance, because the energy continues to be exchanged. Each individual's brain identifies that specific energy as connection with the other individual.

However, when death prohibits the normal energy from being exchanged, the survivor's brain continues to send out a signal to find the lost connection. Instead of connection, the individual finds nothing but emptiness. They send their energy out again and again, but it feels like their energy is being sucked into a black hole. The severed attachment feels like a part of themselves has been amputated. Just like the experience of an amputated limb, the "phantom" feelings of the connection continue long after the energy exchange has been cut. As their energy is drained into nothingness, the grieving individual begins to collapse in on themselves, as if their very being is falling into that black hole of emptiness. The pain of loss experienced as grief is related to this severing of attachment. Flashes of memory of their loved one produce a here-and-now reexperiencing of this process, more energy is drained away, and the internal collapse reoccurs, much like what happens when a trauma memory is triggered.

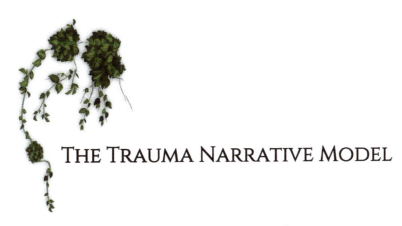

THE TRAUMA NARRATIVE MODEL

How does this Model Address Trauma?

The Trauma Narrative Treatment model is designed to be a brief (six session) method for helping people deal with trauma. The model uses techniques that have been demonstrated through research to be effective, using a creative story entitled *Gold Stone*, which can be easily shared and relates directly to individuals who have experienced trauma. *Gold Stone* addresses the major elements that may be experienced as a result of trauma, including death, profound loss of relationship, life-altering environmental changes, feelings of guilt and self-blame, rage, powerlessness, depersonalization and derealization, loss of a sense of self, dissociation, and spiritual questioning.

Using the story as a reference point, participants in small groups share their personal stories leading up to the trauma. Following along with the main character of the story, participants then share their trauma experiences. Finally, participants begin the process of finding meaning in their experiences, reconnecting with their sense of self to reestablish wholeness, and writing or telling how their story will proceed following the trauma.

The model is designed to be readily implemented by human service-oriented individuals within the community, such as pastors, teachers, community workers, and health workers. One need not be a professional therapist to use this model. The model is a good resource for schools, churches, community organizations, therapists, or other human service workers who need resources to help people with the myriad issues caused by trauma.

Participants identify with the main character from the *Gold Stone* story and relate their experiences to the story character's experiences. Four life stages are stressed: 1) the story of life before the trauma; 2) the story of the traumatic event(s); 3) the story of life since the trauma; and 4) creating and defining their future story. Each lesson has several activities and exercises tied to the storytelling and re-telling process.

Several strong benefits of the model have emerged during our evaluations and research and through use of the model:

1) The model drastically shortens the time needed to provide intervention, from an average of 10-12 or more sessions for brief CBT models to a maximum of 6 sessions;

2) Due to the model's structure and ease of use and training, large numbers of volunteers can be readily trained by a small number of professionals to implement the model;

3) The need for only a few professionals to do the training provides a force multiplier in areas where professional resources are limited, and the immediate need is greater than the available service;

4) The model is a valuable resource for any group or individual dealing with trauma. Schools, churches, missionary groups, and treatment programs have used the model with great success with divorce recovery groups, grief groups, juvenile justice intervention programs, incarceration programs, substance abuse groups, children's homes, trauma groups, and individual counseling for trauma and related issues.

5) The model utilizes a wide range of elements from narrative and trauma research to create a program that addresses the wide variety of issues resulting from trauma, including the immediate shock of the trauma victim, grief and loss, the fragmentation of memory due to trauma, developing meaning from the trauma, religious/spiritual responses to trauma, and the construction of a new narrative for the individual's life (Bowlby, 1980; Herman, 1997; Stewart & Neimeyer, 2007; Van der Kolk, 2014; Meichenbaum, 2017). The following sections review the research that supports our model and explains how and why it works.

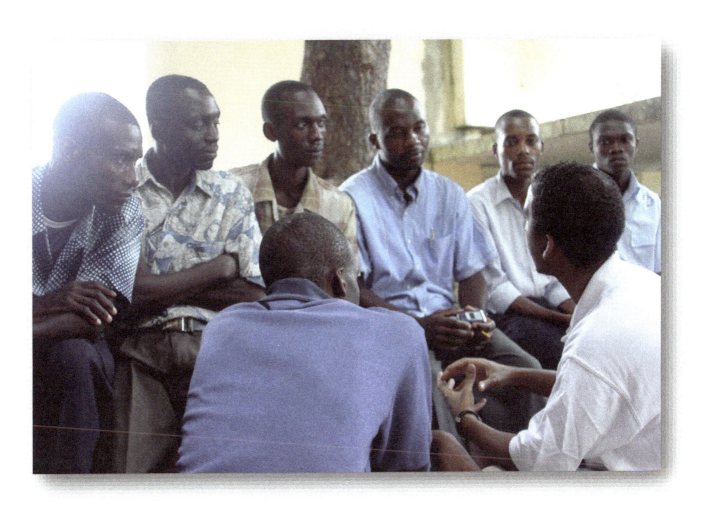

Haitian earthquake survivors share their stories

What does the research say?

Research on the TNT model

In 2010 and 2011, Trauma Narrative Treatment was used in Haiti after the devastating earthquake to train leaders to use the model in their communities. In all, 133 pastors, 85 teachers and paraprofessionals, and 21 Community Workers were trained. The training consisted of a week-long workshop, during which the participants were first treated in small groups using the materials, followed by each individual leading a teaching demonstration of a section of the materials with a small group. The group of 85 in the teacher/paraprofessional workshop volunteered to be assessed with a pre- and post-test using the Davidson Trauma Scale (DTS), a 17-item measure of the symptoms of posttraumatic stress disorder on a four-point frequency and severity scale (Davidson, 1997, 2002). The measure demonstrated a significant decrease in posttraumatic stress scores from the participants after the treatment using the curriculum provided (Lane, et al., 2015). These findings are encouraging.

Since the work in Haiti, groups in Newtown, CT, were trained to use the model after the Sandy Hook School shooting, and the model has been implemented in Rwanda, Dominican Republic, Cambodia, Vietnam, Malaysia, Costa Rica, New Zealand, and in the Middle East. While no pre- and post-research data was collected by these groups, anecdotal reports are equally encouraging on the efficacy of the model.

Other Research used in the model

The model was developed using an integration of a variety of trauma-informed approaches and modalities, based on current research into trauma responses, the specific issues trauma survivors face, and what has been found efficacious in helping ameliorate posttraumatic symptomatology. Based on our research, a narrative base was utilized, combined with mindfulness, breathing, relaxation, body work, movement, spirituality, and expressive therapies such as art and music, presented in a group format to provide a safe, supportive environment and a community with shared experiences.

WHAT IS NARRATIVE?

Stories give form and meaning to our lives, and even substantiate how we understand ourselves (Scheib, 2016). We live and structure our lives around our stories (Madigan, 2010). Our stories have a powerful influence over our memories, behaviors, and identities (Dingfelder, 2008). The central idea of narrative-based therapies is that people make sense of their lives and their worlds through telling stories (Stewart & Neimeyer, 2007; Schauer, Neuner, & Elbert, 2011; Scheib, 2016; Hutto, et al., 2017).

Trauma researchers have noted that developing a coherent narrative is vital for making sense of trauma (Briere & Scott, 2015). From a coherent narrative, the person's identity takes the form of an inner story, complete with setting, scenes, character, plot, and themes, and a beginning, middle, and ending. Life stories are based on biographical facts, but these stories go well beyond the facts as embodied experiences are represented, connecting both past and future to construct stories that make sense to the individual and to their social group (Carless, et al, 2016). This construction and reconstruction of stories helps bring memories to life; how the stories are integrated into life make experiences more or less meaningful (Angus & McLeod, 2004).

REAUTHORING

White & Epston (1990) created narrative therapy, in its reauthoring version, in the late 1980s and early 1990s. Re-authoring has developed into a variety of psychotherapy applications and has become one of the most influential models in the narrative therapies. Reauthoring corrects dysfunctional psychological processes caused by trauma by the construction of new narratives of life.

Trauma causes a problem-saturated narrative which becomes your dominant story and blocks you from alternative ways of thinking, feeling, acting, or behaving. With this powerful dominant story, the individual ignores or forgets other experiences. Cognitive therapists refer to this as cognitive distortion: exaggerated or irrational thought patterns that perpetuate the effects of psychopathological states, especially depression and anxiety (Matos, Santos, Goncalves, & Martins, 2009).

Despite the recurrent and overpowering nature of the dominant story and cognitive distortions, even the most severely traumatized people, White (2007) says, experience what he called "unique outcomes" or stories from their lives that contradict the dominant (trauma) story. The identification and elaboration of unique outcomes (different story lines or narratives) help the individual externalize the trauma and construct new life narratives based on the non-trauma story lines.

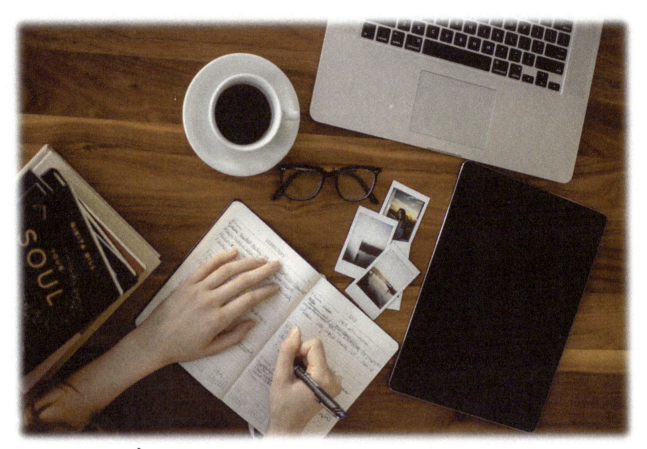

Developing a coherent narrative is vital for making sense of trauma

White and Epson (1990) elaborate a number of techniques giving traumatized individuals possible actions to consider in the development of a new narrative. With this model, it becomes more likely for the trauma survivor to generate options, choose options that are aligned with their values, and engage in those actions that are more successful than the dominant trauma story. As the individual reauthors their story, they are more likely to experience themselves as competent, despite the challenges of the trauma. Through this narrative process, the traumatic event is externalized and loses its power to shape their identity, as the focus shifts to a more internal locus of control as they choose actions effective for handling crisis. They are then in a better position to separate from the traumatic memories that eroded their experience of self (Beaudoin, 2005).

LINGUISTIC REPRESENTATION

Another narrative trauma treatment approach is the Creation of Linguistic Representation. A growing body of research demonstrates that posttraumatic symptoms are a failure of memory; specifically, a disruption in the conversion of sensory experience to verbal or linguistic memory. This concept is important for this model and supports key concepts of narrative therapy. Historical clinical accounts from Janet in the 1880's and 90's noted the fragmented and non-linguistic quality of clients' trauma memories, and more recent studies have demonstrated that traumatic memories are unique, retrieved sensory fragments with no verbal component (Van der Kolk, 2014). Kaminer (2006) further explains:

> Within this literature, the creation of linguistic representation of fragmented images and sensory experiences – that is, the development of a coherent verbal trauma narrative that names and organises the affects, cognitions, behaviours and sensory experiences associated with the trauma – is the central process of recovery for trauma survivors. (pp. 485)

Developments in neurophysiology have added another dimension to the understanding of the narrative processing disruption that identifies traumatic memories (Iacona & Johnson, 2018; Hall, et al., 2018). In the brain in memory creation and storage, the amygdala, part of the limbic system (fight/flight/freeze system), is responsible for interpreting the emotional significance of incoming sensory information. The hippocampus is responsible for integrating and organizing this sensory information and "fitting it into" pre-existing information. This process also includes the pre-frontal cortex in the frontal lobe of the brain and the thalamus in the mid-brain. When trauma occurs, due to the highly emotionally charged nature of trauma memories, hippocampal integration does not occur, not allowing for the inclusion of the contextual time and space that hippocampal integration would allow (Kaminer, 2006). The normally integrated functioning of the amygdala, hippocampus, pre-frontal cortex and thalamus is disrupted, causing fragmentation in the memory and disruption of the conversion of the memory to language (Van der Kolk, 2014).

This research suggests that treatment focusing on developing a coherent trauma narrative is vital to organizing fragmented sensory and emotionally charged memories into narrative linguistic memories (Booker, et al., 2018). Developing this coherent narrative would reduce the intrusive memories and other hallmark symptoms of trauma. Linguistic representation is created by:

1) assisting the person to gradually organize the memory fragments into sequential episodes;

2) helping them identify the characters involved in the story and their actions;

3) helping them identify their emotions, sensations, and thoughts at different stages of the event (Kaminer, 2006). By telling and retelling the story, combined with physical and non-verbal activities, they are able to create linguistic memory and move the memory fragments into a verbal, cohesive memory, thus giving it form and meaning.

Explanatory Account

Another trauma narrative method is to develop an explanatory account. This method helps the traumatized individual develop a cognitively meaningful trauma account. The individual and the group leader or therapist collaborate to reconstruct the trauma story, introducing into the trauma narrative cognitive insights that have been missing. Following a traumatic event, it is very difficult for survivors to develop a cohesive explanatory model of themselves and others that can account for the trauma. Failure to establish this cohesive account means the trauma is unlikely to be integrated into their cognitive map of the world.

An explanatory narrative is developed through exploring the unconscious processes that influence emotions, thoughts, and behaviors. This process helps the individual complete the 'plot' of their life story. Developing a cohesive narrative accounting for their trauma and explaining trauma responses is key for healing.

Posttraumatic Growth

A final theme that emerges in looking at narrative methods of working with trauma is the identification of post-traumatic growth. Post-traumatic growth (PTG) refers to the positive change experienced resulting from the struggle with traumatic or highly stressful life experiences. Reauthoring their trauma story in the context of their preferred values and the societal contributions they have made following their trauma experience is humanizing for the individual and results in PTG (Perdomo, 2018).

The terms, "trauma," "crisis," and "highly stressful events" are often used synonymously when describing this concept. Posttraumatic growth is "manifested in a number of ways or five 'domains of growth' including an increased appreciation of life in general, more meaningful interpersonal relationships, an increased sense of personal strength, changed priorities, and a richer existential and spiritual life" (Tedeschi & Calhoun, 2004).

Since spiritual growth is one of the domains of PTG, Shaw, Joseph, and Linley (2004) conducted a review of eleven empirical studies which examined the relationship between religion, spirituality, and PTG. The authors reported three main findings in their review:

1) studies show that religion/spirituality are usually beneficial to people in dealing with the aftermath of trauma;

2) traumatic experiences can lead to an enrichment or deepening of religion and spirituality;

3) positive religious coping, readiness to face existential questions, religious participation, and religious openness are typically associated with PTG. Tedeschi and Calhoun (2004) suggest that the development of a trauma narrative could either enhance or help facilitate spirituality and PTG. They explain that as traumatized clients experience posttraumatic growth, these changes have a mutual positive influence on their life narrative in general.

Contextually derived master narratives, such as religious or spiritual stories from sacred texts, can support life-giving personal stories and posttraumatic growth (Scheib, 2018). Sacred stories can act as symbolic representations to facilitate reinterpretation of trauma and PTG (Frechette, 2017). Employing spiritually integrated dialogue with trauma survivors facilitates the development of adaptive interpretations of their trauma story (Frechette, 2017). To be effective, the group leader must actively engage with the stories being told, and seek to help the individual develop more coherent, meaningful, and hopeful stories (Scheib, 2018).

When traumatized individuals consider and include the possibility of posttraumatic growth as they reauthor their trauma narratives, they are enabled to develop a revised interpretation of the impact of trauma on their overarching life story. Developing an individual personal life narrative directly influences PTG, and PTG directly influences developing a new life story.

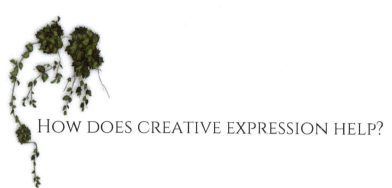

How does creative expression help?

Some experiences cannot be processed verbally, at least not initially. Trauma produces emotional landscapes that are rich canvases for creative expression. Through the use of art, music, writing, and movement, individual and collective creativity promotes sharing and healing (Zerrudo, 2016). Creative expression allows a different part of the traumatized individual's brain to be activated, making access to emotion possible that would otherwise be blocked and promoting connection between the emotional and rational brain. In addition, creative expression is a less threatening way for individuals to share their stories. Human beings are symbolic creatures, and creative expression provides an avenue for symbolic representation of traumatic experiences that individual may be unwilling or unable to share through another mode.

Research on Creative Expression

Studies have demonstrated using written narratives when working with trauma survivors produces an increased depth in emotional experiencing and a decrease in anxiety symptoms (Harrington, et al, 2018). In addition, using creative stories which integrate spirituality can act as symbolic representations of trauma experiences to aide survivors in reinterpreting their trauma in a more adaptive manner (Frechette, 2017).

Research has shown resiliency is increased through creativity and imagination and using the arts to foster creative expression results in decreasing the impact of the trauma event on the individual while increasing resiliency resources. Artistic expression also produced a positive impact on understanding and finding meaning in the trauma event and aids in memory reconsolidation (Hass-Cohen, et al., 2017).

In another study, Carless & Douglas (2016) found writing and sharing creative stories in a group and co-experiencing physical movement along with story-telling allows personal stories of trauma to be shared. The researchers also found that evocative stories of personal trauma are unlikely to be shared in the absence of some embodiment of the experience (i.e., bodily representation, movement, and a sense creating together through various aesthetic forms).

The use of art to create pictorial artifacts aid in regulation processes for traumatized individuals (Gerge & Pedersen, 2017). Another study found integrating art and mindfulness meditation improved emotional self-regulation, communication, imagination, and resiliency (Kalmanowitz & Ho, 2017).

Mindfulness and movement in various forms has been effective in restoring physical regulation, reconnection with the body, and awareness of sensory, body-based feelings (Van der Kolk, 2014). As a result, a sense of self is reestablished. Learning to calm the body through meditation, breathing, and other mindfulness techniques, and learning to remain calm during triggering responses are important steps in recovery from trauma. Physical movement reconnects the trauma survivor to the body, helping them notice how their physical sensations respond to changes in breathing and focus of thoughts. Sensorimotor awareness is essential to healing (Crawford, 2010).

Trauma-sensitive yoga is demonstrated to improve trauma symptomatology, increase resilience, decrease tension, and decrease depression. The mindfulness associated with yoga also improves emotion regulation (Price, et al., 2017). Trauma survivors have an impaired awareness of their physical body and a lack of perception of the connection between environmental stimuli and internal responses. The physical movements associated with yoga, combined with mindfulness exercises, increases body awareness, environmental awareness, and self-awareness. In addition, physical movement requiring body control, accompanied by breathing exercises and mindfulness activities, has been shown to increase tolerance of affective states and improve modulation of physical and affective states dysregulated due to the trauma experience (Rhodes, et al., 2016).

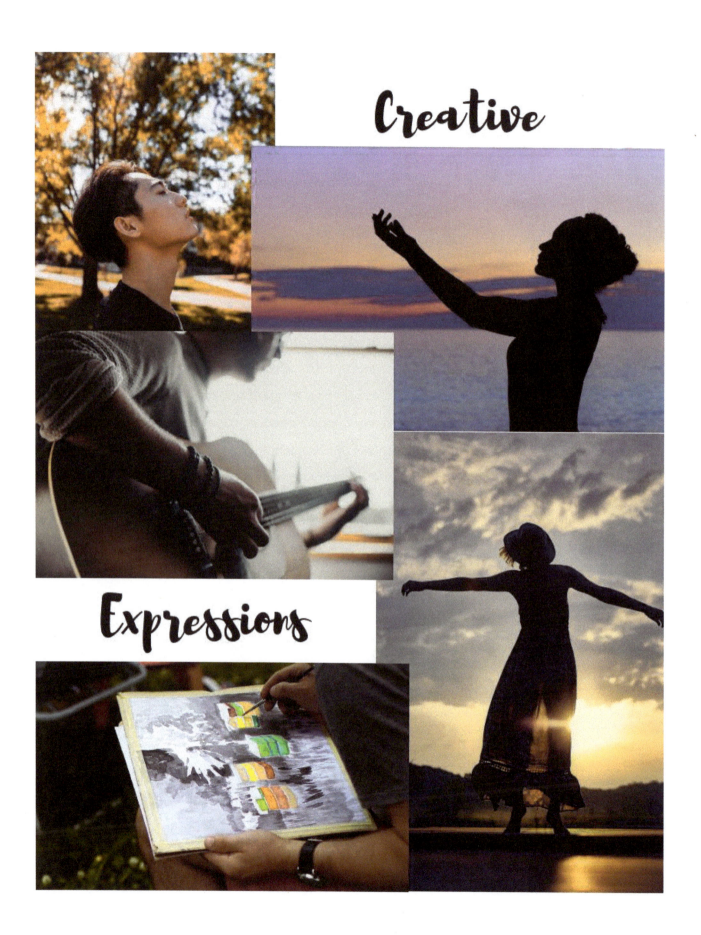

Why Groups?

Groups provide many therapeutic benefits that are not available when working through trauma individually. One of the most positive aspects of working in a group is the built-in supportive community. Human beings are social creatures, and one of the negative consequences of the dissociation resulting from trauma is an inability to attach to others and create workable, satisfying relationships. Hyperreactivity also impedes social functioning. If an individual cannot function as an effective member of a social group, they feel out of sync, isolated, unseen, and unsafe (Van der Kolk, 2014). Research has demonstrated learning to be fully present and engaged with others and becoming a part of a healing community are vital steps to recovery from trauma. Groups provide the opportunity for the traumatized individual to restore their connection to community.

As we have demonstrated, using art, movement, and music, combined with working together with others to create and share stories, produces positive results (Carless & Douglas, 2016). The group provides empathic individuals who can hear trauma stories and who can share related stories of their own trauma, creating a sense of universality, meaning the feeling of not being the only one and knowing others are in the same boat. Group members provide feedback and validation, as each individual shares their story. Groups also offer the opportunity for corrective emotional experiences, catharsis, and interpersonal learning. Safe touch also helps restore connection to the body through sensory integration (Van der Kolk, 2014), and group activities allow for the presence of monitored and structured safe touch.

What remains unspoken to others often cannot be admitted to the self (Van der Kolk, 2014). Trauma is ameliorated when the individual's story is shared within the framework of personal safety and community (Pack, 2008). This process helps survivors find their voice, name their experience, begin to give their experience meaning, integrate their trauma into their life story, and reauthor their stories in such a way they are no longer defined by their trauma.

Leader Skills

The leader has the responsibility for creating an environment of warmth, empathy, and acceptance. These qualities are particularly important for trauma survivors, because their fear (fight/flight/freeze) response is on high alert and trust is often compromised. Group members need to feel they are safe and cared for in their environment to encourage their engagement and openness. How the leader presents and responds is the primary method for establishing that sense of safety and caring. The leader provides a stabilizing presence when he or she is calm, welcoming, understanding, and genuine.

LISTENING

Group members will follow where the leader leads and what the leader models for them. The leader wants group members to offer each other encouragement, support, understanding, genuineness, and unconditional acceptance, so it is important for the leader to model these traits and to establish these types of responses as the expectations for the group. One way the leader can establish this type of warm, open environment is through employing good listening skills. These skills include paying close attention to what each participant is saying, including their nonverbal responses, while demonstrating they are paying attention by making eye contact and avoiding distractions, like taking notes, fidgeting, or looking through materials, and allowing each participant ample time to share. In addition, the leader can demonstrate attending through making reflective statements, which, simply put, are restatements of the gist of what the participant shared, including what it seemed to the leader that the individual was feeling. The following is an example of a reflective response:

    Participant: "I was standing there, you know, watching while the roof of our home collapsed, and I knew my mother and sister were still trapped inside. I just barely made it out myself. I couldn't move. I wanted to run to them, to try to dig them out, but I just couldn't move."

    Leader: "You are saying you felt paralyzed as you watched the roof fall on your mother and sister, and you couldn't do anything to help them. You must've felt so powerless."

    Effective listening assists participants to continue telling their stories, as well as helping them to feel heard and understood. If the leader is unsure what feeling the participant is sharing, he or she can restate the gist of what was shared, then ask, "How did you feel?" to encourage the participant to continue and to share feelings with the group.

QUESTIONING

Through asking effective, open-ended questions, the leader assists group members in continuing the flow of conversation. As long as group members are interacting and sharing, the leader needs to remain attentive and involved, reflecting as needed; however, when the conversation reaches a lull, open-ended questioning can spur participants to further sharing. This is not to say silence in the group is a problem. In fact, moments of silent reflection can be very helpful for participants, so the leader does not want to interrupt those moments with a question. A good leader doesn't feel like he or she must fill all the gaps with chatter. A lull or break in sharing happens when the topic of conversation has run its course and is closing. At those moments, it is helpful for the leader to ask a question that broadens the topic of conversation, or to broach a new topic of conversation followed by a question for participants to consider.

Some examples of open-ended questions are:

What are your thoughts on this topic?

What feelings are stirred up in you when you think about this topic?

How did you feel when (another participant) shared what they shared?

What questions would you like to explore regarding (another participant's) story?

Another form of questioning without actually asking questions, which at times can feel like an interrogation, is to give a directive, such as:

Tell me more about that.

Tell me what was happening that led up to…

Tell me your understanding of what (another participant) just said.

Tell me what you felt when…

Tell me what you're thinking.

Avoid "why" questions, because why questions carry with them a sense of judgment. Focus on what, when, where, and who questions that do not provoke yes or no responses.

At times in groups, some participants share readily, while others are more reticent and quiet. It is up to the leader to draw those quiet participants into the conversation by asking gentle, probing questions or giving directives that express interest in what the quiet participant is thinking and feeling. If the quieter participants still do not want to answer, allow them and all participants the opportunity to decline responding if they are not ready to share. Always be respectful and honoring of all participants.

Another questioning skill is including all group members in every topic by asking for input from the whole group. For example, if one member has just shared a story of loss, the leader could ask, "Do others have a similar experience they would like to share?" or "Has anyone else felt similar feelings to what (another participant) shared?" or "I am very interested in hearing what you were thinking/feeling while (another participant) shared." The leader wants to maximize the benefit of being in a group by fostering whole group participation. The connections made through shared experiences can be a powerful tool for healing, called universality.

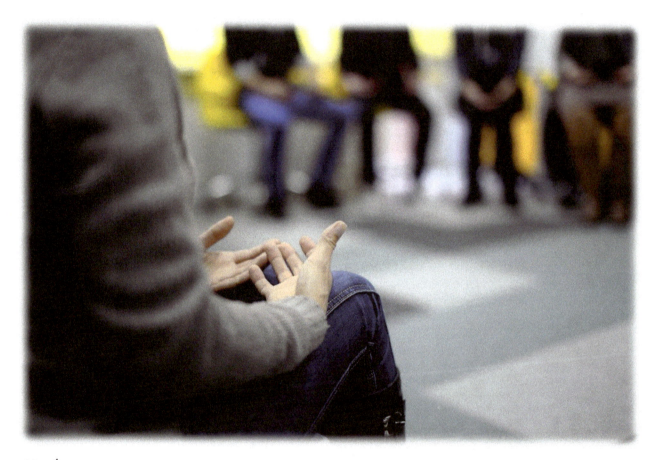

Trauma survivors often share common experiences on the process level, even if their stories are dissimilar.

LINKING

Universality is one of the most powerful therapeutic forces in group. Universality basically provides the benefit of knowing I am not the only one who has experienced something, and we all are in the same boat, so to speak. When trauma occurs, the individual living through the trauma often feels no one could possibly understand what they have gone through or how they feel. It is a very isolating and lonely feeling. Often, trauma survivors do not share their stories for this very reason. In a group, the traumatized individual has the opportunity to share with others who have experienced, if not the same kind of trauma, the same kind of feelings from trauma that he or she is feeling. Those common experiences, when shared, help the trauma survivor to no longer feel isolated and alone. Knowing others share their experience and feel similar feelings offers hope, connection, and relief, and opposes the feeling that something is wrong with them.

Part of the leader's responsibility is to find commonalities or linkages, which are found most often in the feelings and beliefs resulting from trauma. These feelings and beliefs go deeper than the content of the participants' stories; they are found on the process level, meaning the deepest feelings and core beliefs beneath the content of their stories.

Process issues are what makes things "tick." Consider a clock. On the surface of the clock, we see the time is 10:58 am. What all came together for the clock to say 10:58 am? All the gears and mechanisms and weights and springs within the clock drove the hands to say 10:58. So, no matter what the numbers are on the clock face, the gears and mechanisms within the clock work the same way. In this analogy, 10:58 is the content, and the internal workings are the process. Another way to think about it is that what you are seeing and hearing from the participants are symptoms. The leader's responsibility is to understand and conceptualize what all the underlying issues are that are causing and driving those symptoms. The symptoms are the content, and what drives the symptoms is the process.

Trauma survivors often share common experiences on the process level, even if their stories are dissimilar. Some of those common *feelings* include paralyzing fear, feeling overwhelmed, a feeling of disconnection or numbness, powerlessness, feeling trapped, feeling worthless, feeling to blame, and feeling shameful. Some of the common *beliefs* coming from trauma include it is my fault, I am bad, I am tainted, I don't matter, I am unloved, I am unwanted, I'm not good enough, I am sick, I am damaged goods, everything is out of control, and I will never be okay. Using reflection and questioning skills, the leader can explore these common feelings and beliefs and draw linkages between group members who share similar experiences on the process level.

Forming a linkage would look something like the following example:

Participant 1: Ever since we lost our home, I have felt completely ungrounded, like I am missing an anchor or something. It is like I lost who I am somewhere, and I can't seem to find it again.

Leader: Has anyone else in the group ever felt like they lost themselves?

Participant 2: Oh, definitely. My entire childhood, I was told I was nothing. My father would beat me and call me a failure, stupid, worthless, no good. That's who I believed I was. I still believe it to this day.

Leader: So, (participant 2), you basically lost yourself from the start.

Participant 2: I don't think I've ever known myself.

Leader: It sounds like you and (participant 1) have something in common, that feeling of losing yourself. Does anyone else share similar feelings?

The more group members the leader can link to a process feeling or belief, the stronger the therapeutic force of universality. Cohesion, defined as bonds created among group members, within the group grows deeper and relationships between group members grow stronger, maximizing the benefit of the group.

Refocusing

Another responsibility of the group leader is to maintain the vision and purpose of the group in the forefront at all times. Sometimes the group can lose focus and get off track. For example, a group member can get caught up in telling their story and can begin to share other stories with little or no relevance to their trauma experience or the experiences of other group members. During those times, the group leader can gently refocus the group by giving a directive or asking a question leading back to the main topic. The leader does not need to interrupt any group member in their sharing; instead, the leader can interject during a pause, turn to other group members, and ask their feelings regarding what the participant just shared, or ask an open-ended question that bring back the topic being originally discussed.

Because this model provides a structure for the group meetings, it is easy for the leader to refocus the group by simply moving to the next question for discussion. Keeping the group on track and maintaining structure assists trauma survivors in feeling safe and secure in the group. The leader must keep in mind that trauma survivors respond to feeling out of control with heightened anxiety. Because of this heightened anxiety, some group members, in the absence of leader intervention, may feel the need to control the group themselves, which ultimately leaves the group, including the member or members trying to control, feeling out of control. It is important, therefore, for the leader to maintain the structure and flow of the group meeting according to the manual description; however, the leader does not need to add to the anxiety of the group by attempting to control in response to his or her own anxiety or feeling like he or she needs to make something happen. Provide the structure, maintain the flow, and allow the group to unfold.

Imparting Information

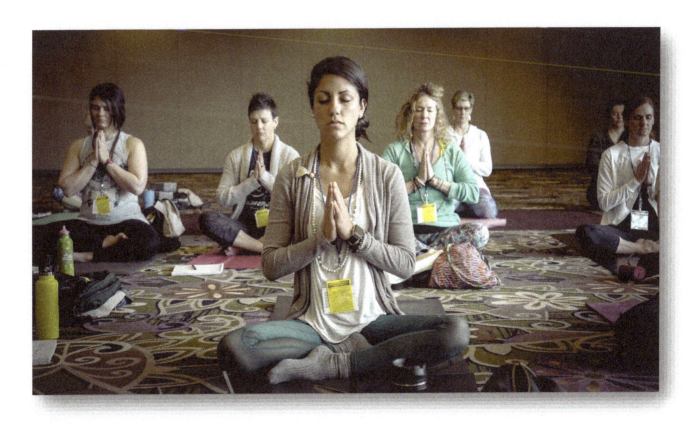

Teaching new information is an important role for the group leader

At times, the group leader will take on a didactic role. For example, when leading group members in a breathing exercise or movement exercise, the leader will need to teach group members how to do the exercise through explanation and demonstration. Teaching is an important role for the group leader. Leaders need to take care, however, to not separate themselves as superior to or above/over group members. Establishing a hierarchy within the group can undermine group cohesion and group process, as group members begin to look to the leader to tell them what to say or how to feel. This is not the function of the group leader, largely because the leader is not the expert on the participants' lives, so the leader needs to maintain the position of sharing the group experience with the group members, coming alongside them on their journey.

ASSESSING NEED

One of the most important skills for a leader of this particular model is the ability to assess if participants need a higher level of care than can be provided in this type of group. This model focuses on sharing stories, first through looking at the story of the main character in the book, *Gold Stone,* then through participants sharing their personal stories as they draw connections between their stories and the story presented in *Gold Stone*. However, the leader needs to always be aware of the responses of the participants to sharing their stories. If a group member appears to become severely agitated, deeply distressed, or disengaged completely, as if they are mentally somewhere else, the leader needs to intervene with that group member. First, the leader can try a re-centering exercise, such as grounding the participant in their body by having them focus on the feeling of their feet on the floor, their back against the chair, and the breath coming in and out of their lungs. The leader can ask all group members to participate in a relaxation exercise, including slow, deep breathing, and tightening and releasing muscle groups. However, if the group member is unable to participate in these activities, the leader needs to say to the group, "We are going to take a break for a few minutes," and gently escort the struggling member out of the group.

If a member needs to separate from the group, one of the leaders needs to stay with that group member. Have the group member focus on and describe their surroundings to reorient them to the present. Talk about safe topics for the group member, topics the leader knows the member has been able to discuss easily, such as work, extracurricular activities, hobbies, etc. Allow the group member as much time as they need to calm and re-center themselves.

Once the member is completely calm and states they are ready, the leader may have a conversation with the member to assess if they are able to return to the group. If the member is hesitant to return or feels the experience was too distressing for them, the leader can suggest another, more appropriate level of care, such as individual counseling. The leader needs to be encouraging and positive with the group member, urging the participant to pursue their own best interests only and reassuring them it is not a failure to leave the group if it does not meet their needs.

However, if the group member believes they are benefitting from the group and they desire to return, the leader may still ask the group member to give themselves additional time to recover from their response to the session before returning. In fact, the leader may be more realistic about what the participant can handle than the participant themselves. So, reassure the participant that there is no urgency for either the participant or the leader to return, and do not allow the group member to rush themselves.

INSTILLATION OF HOPE

Another powerful therapeutic force in group is the instillation of hope. Simply joining a group brings some level of hope to the participants, as they have taken the first step toward healing. The leader can foster instillation of hope in the group by bringing their own hope for the participants' healing to the first meeting. If the leader believes healing is not only possible but believes it will come through the experience of this model and beyond, the group members are likely to also feel hope for themselves.

One way to help instill hope is to periodically take a step back and examine progress that has been made during the group. The leader can point out changes he or she has observed in group members through the process, draw parallels from one session to the next to demonstrate growth, and encourage participants to observe changes and growth in one another.

Having a commencement or graduation ceremony at the end of the model is a good way to close the group with a sense of hope in their future. Group members are encouraged by feeling they have successfully completed the model. A final ceremony could also allow group members to give each other positive feedback and encourage each other to continue to use the skills they have learned as they leave the group.

Design the ending ceremony to reflect the way the group has worked together during their experience. Symbolic rituals are meaningful and assist group members in taking metaphorical "gifts" with them as they leave the group. Some examples of ending activities include: having group participants create their own symbolic representation of their group, like a group drawing or sculpture; giving each group member a small box, then having group members write something they will always remember about, or something they learned from, each other on a slip of paper to be placed in each members' gift box; having each group member stand before the group, share something they will take away from their group experience, and receive a certificate of "graduation." The leader could also ask the group to design their own ceremonial experience as part of the ending process. Allow the participants to be creative in how they want to express their feelings about the end of their group experience.

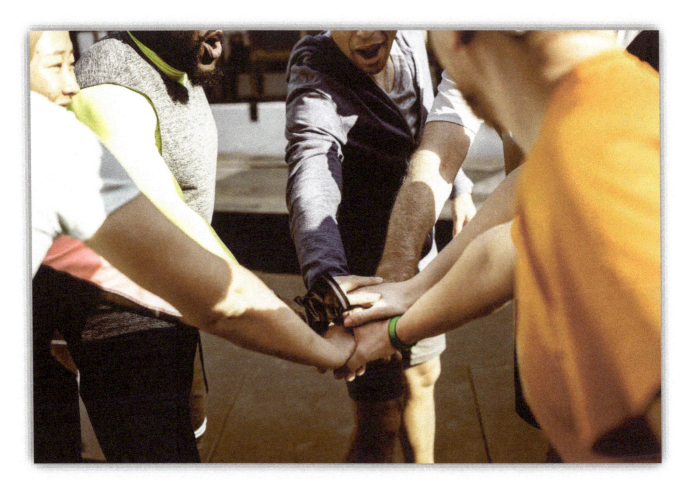

Each group develops their own closing ceremony to instill hope for success as they move forward

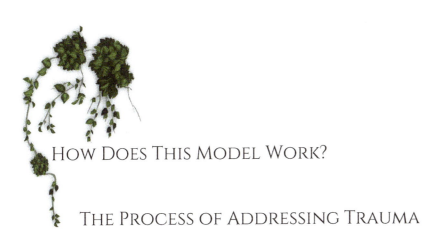

How Does This Model Work?

The Process of Addressing Trauma

Having learned the effects, results, and symptoms associated with trauma, and looked at some of the research on narrative combined with creative expression in addressing trauma, we will now discuss the process that we will use to help trauma survivors recover from their traumatic experience. The process includes: learning to center themselves in the body, to calm and focus their mind, and to remain connected to their mind and body even when talking about their trauma; learning to be fully present in the here-and-now and to remain connected with others; learning to give language to their story and to integrate their trauma story into their overarching life story; learning to give meaning to their trauma experience as an integral part of their life story and re-authoring their story with an ending of their choosing.

The trauma survivor can retrain their body and its paralyzed fixation in fight/flight/freeze response by the way they breathe and move. Meditation and/or prayer, music and movement to music, and deep breathing and relaxation exercises are all excellent methods of retraining the arousal system (Crawford, 2010). At the same time, body and mind connection can be achieved through mindfulness, meaning paying attention to bodily responses to the here-and-now environment, noting those responses are temporary and ever-changing, and observing how the body responds to intentional breathing and movement. While paying attention to bodily responses, the traumatized individual can notice also how their thoughts and emotions interact, and how their thoughts and emotions are experienced in your body. This process helps the individual remember or perhaps realize for the first time that they are in charge of themselves – their body and their mind. Restoring agency is key to trauma recovery.

Because this program is designed for groups, the important need for establishing connections with healing relationships in a supportive environment is addressed. Research has demonstrated that a support network is one of the most powerful predictors for successful resolution of trauma (Van der Kolk, 2014). All individuals are wired for relationship, meaning we are meant to connect with and depend on each other. This basic wiring is subverted because of trauma and needs to be reestablished. Group process allows for connection to be reestablished in a safe, supportive social context.

Part of rediscovering a sense of self involves activating the part of the brain that connects the rational brain with the emotional brain, which lets the individual be aware of themselves. Translating the trauma experience into language, writing to access their inner world, drawing a memory picture while attending to the bodily and emotional responses that result, and sharing through language their inner experiences of how they are responding to the sharing of others can all help access the self-awareness seat in their brain. Having others attend in a caring and compassionate way to the individual's story helps keep them connected to their emotional brain and helps minimize re-traumatization through retelling.

Finally, giving meaning to their experience allows the traumatized individual to incorporate the trauma as part of their overarching story and allows them to re-author the ending of their story according to their own choices and desires. Part of this process is realizing, by integrating the trauma into their life story, that they are not defined by the trauma; in other words, their personhood or nature existed before the trauma and continues to exist after the trauma. *Gold Stone,* the story we use as a backdrop for the telling of their stories, brings this point to life. The story includes trauma experiences and multiple losses and offers symbolic representations of spiritual elements to facilitate finding meaning and reinterpretation of their trauma in an adaptive manner (Frechette, 2017). *Gold Stone* provides a master narrative which can support developing life-giving personal narratives (Scheib, 2016).

How to Use This Model

The story of the *Gold Stone* and the following exercises and activities are designed to be used with small groups by a counselor, teacher, pastor, lay-counselor, or volunteer support person. If the group approach is not possible, the leader may implement the program with individuals. The objectives of the story of the *Gold Stone* and the supporting activities are to help people deal with the residual effects of trauma. The difficulties they are having may range from experiencing grief, being fearful, having nightmares, being easily startled or frightened by loud or unusual noises, or reporting that they want or need some help with the bad memories. Anyone reporting difficulty of this type may benefit from participation in these groups or from individual intervention using these materials.

The program is designed to last for six sessions. It is advisable to let some time elapse between sessions. Our research has shown that spending longer times with these activities allows greater time for the concepts and personal implications to be reflected upon and internal changes to take place (Lane, et al., 2015, 2017). We recommend spreading the sessions over a minimum of three weeks (two meetings per week) or a maximum of six weeks (one meeting per week with follow up small group activities and homework between meetings).

The key to presenting this program is to actively engage the participants through drawing, speaking, writing, movement, and other learning activities included here. When using the model with children and youth, it is important to make parents and caregivers aware of the goals of this program and ways they may help. Solicit support by explaining the program to them and encouraging them to ask their child about the story and the activities they are doing.

It is important for the leader to employ active listening as the participants share. Allow adequate time after questions are posed for contemplation prior to sharing, and permit periods of silence for processing and integration; do not feel as if every moment must be filled with discussion or activity.

Because of the nature of responses to trauma, someone in the group may experience emotional dysregulation during a session. Should that occur, the leader would need to suspend continuing with the activity or discussion going on at that time, and assist the individual with calming through breathing, mindfulness activities, and slow, gentle movements. Have the individual gently tap their body in time and sway with soft, rhythmic music. If possible, have a small tray of soft or kinetic sand available for the individual to touch and squeeze. A small lump of clay could also be used. Encourage them to slow and regulate their breathing, and to attend to their bodily responses and movements. Have them notice each part of their body and how it feels against their seat, the floor, the arms of their chair, the back of their chair, etc. During this time, the rest of the group may also practice their mindfulness exercises and relaxation, because the more they practice, the more in tune and connected they become. When the individual reports feeling calm and regulated, the leader may resume the discussion or activity.

Overview of a Typical Session

Small groups work best when there are no less than six and no more than ten group members, including the leader or co-leaders. Arrange the group so that everyone can see and hear well. Circles or semicircles work best if the space and the layout of the meeting area allows. The circle/ semicircle allows everyone to see everyone else, and group members can be encouraged to look at who is talking and listen attentively when others are talking. Each group should take a minimum of one hour and a maximum of ninety minutes. A typical session proceeds as follows:

1. <u>Review the previous lesson</u>.

In the case of the first lesson, give an introduction and an overview. For later lessons, when reviewing, ask open-ended questions, such as "Who can tell me what we've learned so far?" or "Someone tell us what the story was about." When homework has been assigned between sessions, review and discuss the homework.

2. <u>Reinforce</u>.

Ask the group if they have been thinking about what they have learned so far. Reinforce and encourage those who demonstrate that they are thinking about these lessons and who are beginning to demonstrate a better understanding of the issues associated with the traumatic events in the *Gold Stone* story or their own story.

3. <u>Introduce the activities for today</u>.

Each lesson has activities associated with the lesson that have a specific objective. State the objective to the group members. For example: "Today we are going to look at *Caonaciba's* life before the traumatic event. We are also going to explore what life was like for us before our traumatic event." Instruct the group members to pay close attention to what life was like before the trauma for the story character and for each group member. Ask questions and make statements that lead to introspection, such as, "Notice what/ how you feel when…" and "What do you feel while…?" Also lead members to explore the narrative by asking, "What happens next?"

4. <u>Present the section of the story</u>.

Read the part of the story, *Gold Stone*, appropriate to the lesson, pausing occasionally to ask questions and assist with understanding.

5. <u>Review the part of the story</u>.

Follow the questions in the lesson for that day's activities. In addition, ask the group members Who, What, When, Where, and How questions about the story to reinforce the ideas and build comprehension of the story. This reinforces the building of a cohesive narrative with a beginning, a middle, and an ending, an important piece of resolving their own trauma.

6. <u>Summarize</u>.

Review the main points of the part of the story you covered today, and tie those back to the main points of previous sections of the story. Be sure to highlight succinctly all the main points you have covered in all the lessons.

7. <u>Transition to the activity</u>.

Introduce the activity which reinforces the concept for today. Complete the activity or activities according to the instructions.

8. <u>Wrap up</u>.

Bring the group together to review, highlight, and reinforce the ideas and concepts covered by the activity, and to discuss the relationship of the activity to the concepts.

9. <u>Preview</u>.

Tell the group what the lesson will be next time and encourage them to apply the ideas and concepts of the lessons they have completed so far. Encourage the group members to talk with their loved ones (family members, friends, or support systems) about the story and the lessons. Assign any homework that is prescribed by that section of the materials.

After the lesson, think through how the lesson went, what the strengths and weaknesses were, how to improve the next lesson, and ways you can demonstrate the concepts for the group members. Between and during lessons, if possible, monitor the group members closely for any trauma symptoms, point out ways that individuals are incorporating the exercises and information well, and encourage those who may still be having some difficulty.

Keep the *Gold Stone* book available for the group to use as necessary. Some group members may wish to re-read the book on their own. You will use this story as a reference point to complete the exercises for all group meetings.

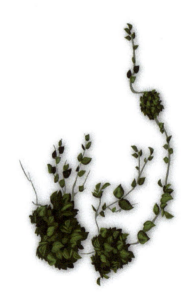

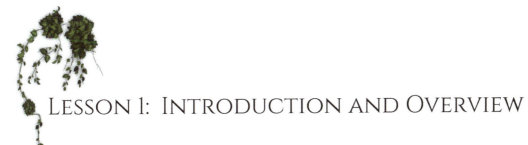

Lesson 1: Introduction and Overview

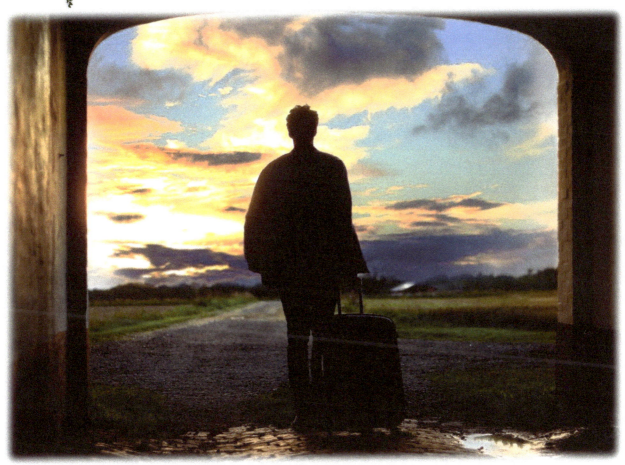

Your journey toward restoration begins

Supplies needed: The book, *Gold Stone,* Paper (butcher paper, sketch pads, printer paper, etc.), crayons, colored pencils, or colored markers, music player, soothing and rhythmic music selections.

The leader greets each group member and introduces him/herself. Then each member introduces him/herself. The leader then explains the purpose of the group and what will be happening for the next six meetings.

Have everyone stand up, remaining in the circle. Play soft, slow, and rhythmic instrumental music in the background during the exercise. Ask the members to breathe deeply, concentrating on how their body feels as the air enters their lungs, and then how their body feels as the air leaves their lungs. Have members focus on breathing as deeply and slowly as possible. Next, ask them to focus on their exhale, taking a pause for a beat after each exhale. Once again, ask members to notice how their body feels, suggesting they check in on each part of their body.

Explain the purpose of the exercise to members by saying, "We are going to notice our breathing today, because if we are feeling our breaths entering and leaving our bodies, we are connected to our bodies in the here-and-now, because we can breathe in the present, but we cannot breathe in the past or future." Take just a few moments and allow anyone who wants to share how this exercise felt to share.

Divide the group into dyads and give each member a piece of butcher paper long enough for them to lie down on and a set of markers to share. Have each dyad take turns drawing an outline around each other while they are lying on their butcher paper. Make sure everyone is respectful of any boundaries set by the individual being drawn (for example, if the individual prefers they are not touched by the marker or the tracer's hand, or if there are certain places the individual wants the tracer to avoid completely, have the tracer fill in those sections once the individual stands).

Then, ask the members to draw on their "body" outline where they feel their feelings. They can use different colors and different symbols to represent the feelings, or simply draw how it feels to them and where each feeling is located. For members that struggle with identifying feelings or locating those feelings in their body, remind them of the breathing exercise and suggest they begin with how they felt after the deep breathing. Suggest they explore the basic emotions of happy, sad, mad, and scared, if they struggle to name any feelings.

Instruct the dyads to share their drawings with each other once both have finished the exercise. For each area of the body identified in the drawing, have the partners ask each other, "If that part of your body could speak, what would it say?" Once the sharing is complete, instruct members to ask each other to notice how their bodies are feeling now, and to share any differences they sense than when they started the exercise. Then, allow any members who would like to share with the whole group to share their drawings. (Kaduson and Schaefer, 2003).

After the introduction and initial body awareness exercises, the leader reads the book, *Gold Stone,* aloud to the group. After reading the story, the leader asks Who, What, When, Where, and How questions to make sure the group members understand the story and can report back the significant characters, events, ideas, and concepts.

Next, ask the group to draw their favorite character or event in the story, share it with a partner, and explain why they like that person or event most. In order to build group cohesion, it is a good idea to have members pair up with someone new rather than remaining in their initial dyad; however, if someone expresses discomfort with changing partners, be flexible and allow members to operate within their comfort level. Ask for volunteers to share with the whole group.

After the sharing and discussion, as time allows in the first session, tell the group you want them to make two more drawings. The first is called "**This is Me: I Am…**". It is their self-portrait. It should be a picture of how they see themselves. Once again, members can use symbolic representations. Encourage those who feel insecure with their drawings that as long as the picture expresses their feelings and internal view of themselves, and they feel connected to it, then the drawing is exactly what it needs to be.

The second is "**My Space**." This drawing shows how they see their world, their position in it, and their reaction to it. Use the following questions to guide the exercise: Do you believe you have a space in your world? What are your relationships with significant others? Where do your fears, wishes, anger, depression, and personal strengths and weakness fit in? How do you tolerate your world in the present? Do you feel isolated and withdrawn or included and part of the world around you? (Spring 1993). Once again, encourage those members who feel uncomfortable with art that the exercise is for their benefit, and it only matters how they view the questions and how they represent their own feelings on the paper.

After each drawing, discuss the drawings and what they mean to the members. If time does not allow for completing this exercise during the first session, assign the two drawings as homework, then have the discussion on the two drawings at the start of the next session.

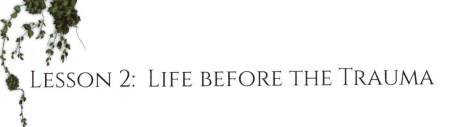

Lesson 2: Life before the Trauma

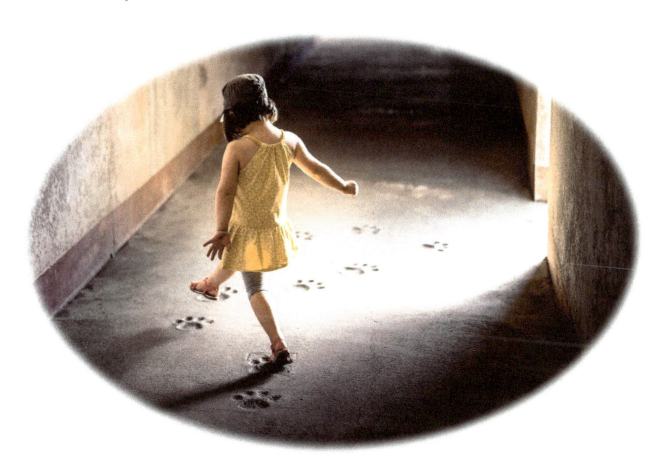

tracing

your

steps

Supplies needed: The book, *Gold Stone,* music player, soothing and rhythmic music selections

Greet everyone and ask if there are any questions before getting started. Once questions have been addressed, tell the group that for this meeting, you will be looking at life before the trauma. Tell them you hope that everyone will feel comfortable enough to share their own story.

Have the group retell the story of *Gold Stone*. Listen carefully and ask questions to reinforce the concepts, themes, and main ideas of the story and to make sure they sequence the story correctly, with a beginning, a middle, and an ending. Prompt members with questions such as, "And then what happened?" or "What happened next in the story?" Encourage as many group members as possible to contribute to the retelling of the story.

Pre-Trauma History and Identity

Read Part I of the story (pages 1-9) and have the group reflect on Caonaciba's life before the trauma.

Ask and discuss the following questions:

    Who was he?

    What was his life like?

    What were some of his beliefs?

    What were some of his values?

    What was his reality?

Then, shift to a discussion of the participants' lives. Ask the following questions:

How are you like Caonaciba?

Reflect on your life before your traumatic event.

Who were you?

What was your life like?

What were your beliefs?

What were your values?

What was your reality?

Have each person share their reflections and have the group discuss them. Be attentive, kind, and supportive and encourage all the group members to listen attentively and support the other members as they share. Reinforce appropriate behavior and thank each person as they share by letting them know that you understand how hard it can be to talk about difficult personal things.

Once everyone has had the chance to share their reflections, have everyone stand and complete the deep breathing exercise again. Play soft, slow, and rhythmic music in the background. This time, as they are breathing, add simple movements. Remind members to continue to notice their breathing, to focus on exhaling and pausing before inhaling again, and to notice how each part of their body feels. The simple movements can be swaying gently, lifting their arms with their palms facing each other from their sides to above their heads and stretching toward the sky, extending their arms out to the sides with palms down, or spreading their feet apart slightly and shifting their weight from foot to foot in rhythm with the music. Make sure during their movements they are still focused on feeling their breaths enter and leave their bodies, and they are keeping their breathing slow, deep, and steady. Check in with members and allow them to share how this exercise felt. Ask them to compare their feelings during this exercise with the last breathing exercise. Finally, point out how their feelings within their body change with each movement and ask them to notice the changes.

If supplies are readily available and time allows, once the breathing and movement exercise is complete, have three stations set up in the room:

1) a plastic tray half-filled with art sand, play sand, or kinetic sand;
2) a plastic sheet with a lump or two of clay; and/or
3) a can of shaving cream and paper towels or cloths.

If these supplies are not available, go directly to the homework. If some or all of these supplies are available, divide the group into dyads, and allow the dyads to take turns at each of the stations. The instruction for each station is to immerse their hands in the material and notice how it feels against their skin. For the sand, run your fingers through the sand and move the sand around in the tray. For the clay, knead the clay and form it and shape it with your hands. For the shaving cream, spread shaving cream on your hands and massage it with your fingers into your hands and (if comfortable) arms.

Have the dyads share with each other what they notice about how the material feels against their skin and how their bodies react to the touch of the materials. Remind members to keep their breathing slow and deep as they work with the materials. Once everyone has had the opportunity to experience each of the materials, check in with members and allow anyone to share with the whole group who would like to share.

Once the breathing and sensory exercises are completed, share the following homework exercise for them to complete before the next meeting:

Homework: Have each person write or draw or tell their story of life before the trauma. Tell them they will share the story of their life before the trauma for the next lesson. Encourage the group members to work on their story with their loved ones (family members, friends, or support systems) at home.

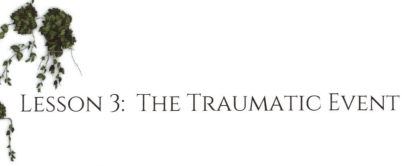

Lesson 3: The Traumatic Event

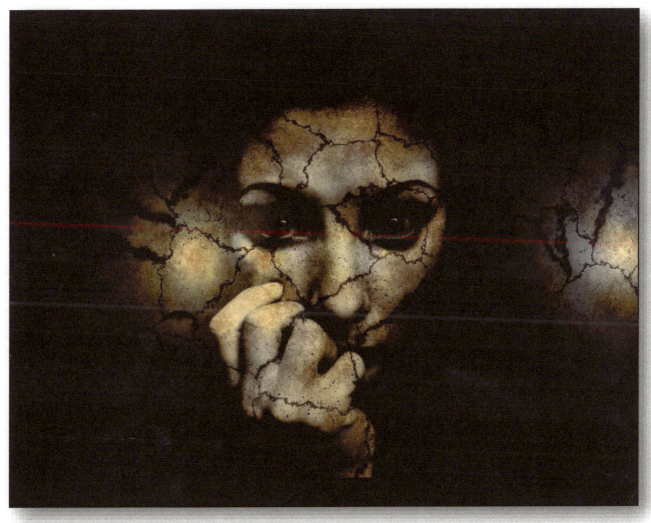

Trauma fractures your perceptions and your sense of self

Supplies needed: the book, *Gold Stone*, your pre-prepared butterfly, cardboard, construction paper, tape, notebook or printer paper, crayons, colored pencils, markers, pens, pencils, music player, soothing and rhythmic music selections

Greet everyone and ask if there are any questions before getting started. Once questions have been addressed, ask each person to share their homework by reading aloud, sharing their drawing, or telling their story of life before the trauma. After processing the homework, ask the group to review the previous portions of the story by asking, "Who can share with me what has happened in the story so far?" After a brief review, begin this lesson.

The Trauma and its Effects

Read Part II (pages 11-15) of Caonaciba's story and have the group reflect on his trauma.

Ask and discuss the following questions:

What happened to Caonaciba?

How do you think he felt?

How did his life change?

What happened to his beliefs?

What happened to his values?

What happened to his reality?

Then, shift to a discussion of the participants' lives. Ask the following questions:

How are you like Caonaciba?

Reflect on your trauma.

What happened to you?

How did you feel?

How did life change?

What happened to your beliefs?

What happened to your values?

What happened to your reality?

Have each person share their reflections and have the group discuss them. Be attentive, kind, and supportive and encourage all the members to listen attentively and support the others as they share. Reinforce appropriate behavior and thank each person as they share by letting them know that you understand how hard it can be to talk about difficult personal things. Then transition into the following large group activity:

The Message (modified from an activity first presented by Cindy A. Stear, in Kaduson and Schaefer, 2003).

Before the activity begins, the group leader creates a large, colorful butterfly from available materials such as construction paper, cardboard, and tissue paper. Tape the butterfly on the wall in the room. To begin the activity, the leader shares that one of the difficult things that happens when we lose someone is that we feel we do not have the chance to say goodbye, or to say other things to our loved ones we wanted to say. Explain to the group that the butterfly represents new life, since it begins life as a caterpillar, then goes into a cocoon (which is like death) and is reborn out of the cocoon as a new and beautiful butterfly. The leader continues, "So, we are going to use this butterfly to carry a message to any loved ones that we have lost."

Have the group members draw pictures, write poems, write letters, or create their own way to communicate their message for their loved ones. While they are creating their messages, play soft, slow, and rhythmic music in the background. If some members are unable to verbalize what they want to say, or if they seem to struggle with expressing these feelings, the leader can suggest they draw a picture of themselves doing their favorite activity with their loved ones or draw a picture that represents their feelings they are having about their loss.

Once the messages are completed, have the group members tape the drawing or writing onto the butterfly. Inform the group the butterfly will take their messages to their loved ones that evening. Ask the group what they believe their loved ones will say in response to their messages. Ask members to notice how their bodies feel as they share. Once everyone who wants to share has done so, allow the group to create a solemn ceremony to signify the messages are ready and to prepare the butterfly to go on its way. Allow the group to determine how they want to perform their ceremony and what it will include. Allow creative expression based on what is meaningful to the group.

After the group ends and the members have gone home, the leader removes the butterfly from the room so the next meeting day, the group members may notice that it is gone.

Once the exercise is completed, share the following homework exercise for them to complete before the next meeting:

Homework: Have each person write or draw or tell their story of their traumatic experience. Tell them they will share the story of their experience for the next lesson. Encourage the members to do this assignment with their loved ones (family members, friends, or support system).

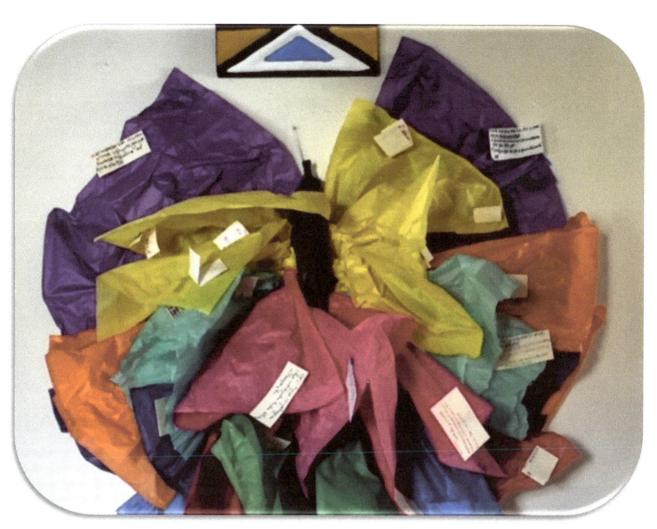

A completed butterfly activity from a group in Rwanda

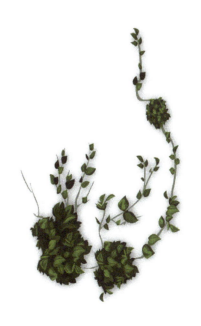

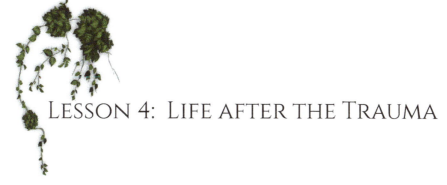

Lesson 4: Life after the Trauma

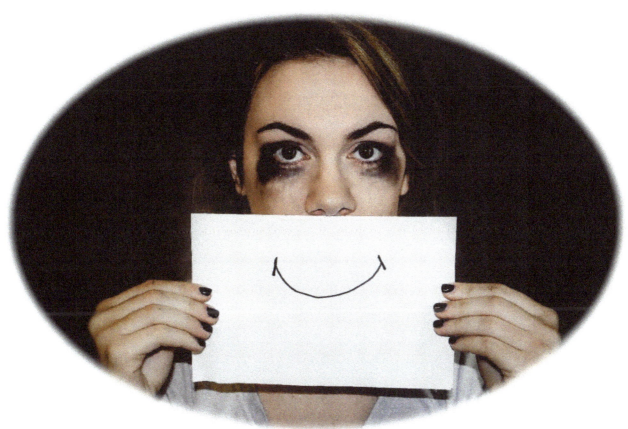

Mired in the trauma reliving it each time the memory is triggered

Supplies needed: the book, *Gold Stone*, notebook or printer paper, crayons, colored pencils, markers, pens, pencils, music player, soothing and rhythmic music selections

Greet everyone and ask if there are any questions before getting started. Once questions have been addressed, ask each person to share their homework by reading aloud, sharing their drawing, or telling their story of their trauma. Notice anyone who is able to connect with feelings as they tell their trauma story and allow ample time for the expression and sharing of those feelings, as members are able to share. If they are unable to find language to share their feelings, provide paper and crayons or markers and suggest they draw out those feelings for themselves. Ask them to focus on where the feelings are occurring in their bodies. Encourage and reinforce the decision to share their trauma experience with others. Once everyone has had opportunity to share and discuss the homework, ask the group to review the previous portions of the story by asking, "Who can share with me what has happened in the story so far?" After a brief review, begin this lesson.

The Impact of the Trauma on My Story

Read Part III (pages 17-21) of Caonaciba's story and reflect on the impact of the trauma on his story.

Ask and discuss the following questions:

What happened to Caonaciba after the traumatic event?

What was his life like after the trauma?

What happened to his beliefs?

What happened to his values?

What was his reality now?

Then, shift to a discussion of the participants' lives. Ask the following questions:

How are you like Caonaciba?

Reflect on your life since the trauma.

What is happening in your life now?

How do you feel?

What is life like for you now?

What happened to your beliefs?

What happened to your values?

What is your reality now?

Have each person share their reflections and have the group discuss them. Be attentive, kind, and supportive and encourage all the members to listen attentively and support the others as they share. Reinforce appropriate behavior and thank each person as they share by letting them know that you understand how hard it can be to talk about difficult personal things. Once everyone has had the opportunity to share, transition to the following activity.

The Rhythm of Life

Begin by playing slow, soothing, rhythmic instrumental music. Have members stand and do the deep breathing exercise they have practiced during previous lessons. After about five slow, deep breaths, ask members to notice the rhythm of the music that is playing. Then ask members to begin tapping along with the music's rhythm. They may tap lightly against their legs, gently clap their hands together, or gently tap with their fingers against their chest. Remind members to continue to pay attention to their breathing as they tap with the rhythm of the music, noticing each breath as it enters and leaves their body.

Pay attention to any members who are having difficulty with finding the rhythm of the music and encourage and assist them as needed. Instruct members that the goal is not to make loud noise with their tapping or clapping, but to gently synchronize themselves with the rhythm of the music. Ask them to notice how their bodies feel as they get in tune with the music's rhythms. Once the activity is completed, discuss and allow members to share how they felt during the activity. Then, as time allows, transition to the next exercise.

My Life's Road

Have members draw a timeline of their lives, including significant events and any things that have shaped their lives. Encourage members to be creative in how they express these events and how they choose to create their unique personal timeline. Play slow, soft, and rhythmic music in the background as members are working on the exercise. Ask for volunteers to share their drawing. Discuss the drawings and what they mean.

Once the exercise is completed, share the following homework exercise for them to complete before the next meeting.

Homework: Have each person write or draw or tell their story of life after the trauma. Tell them they will share the story of their life since the trauma for the next lesson. Encourage the group members to do this assignment with their loved ones (family members, friends, or support system).

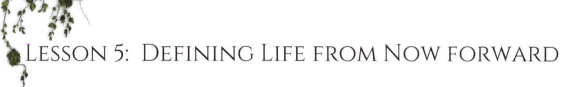

Lesson 5: Defining Life from Now Forward

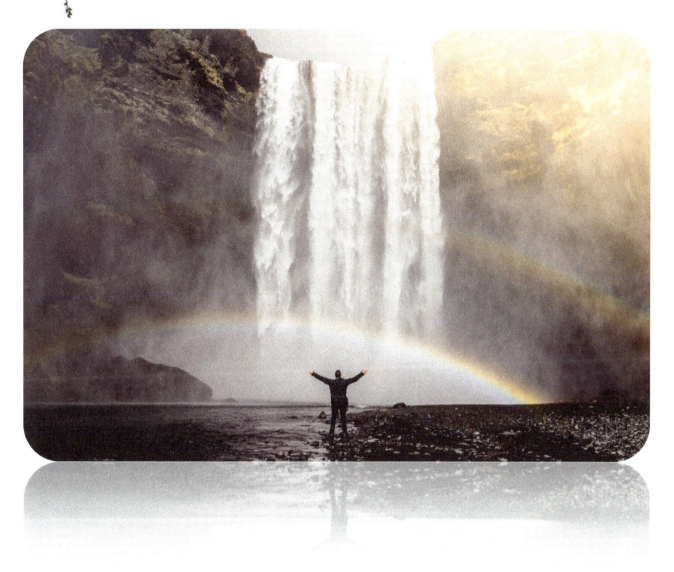

Your trauma does not define you

Supplies needed: the book, *Gold Stone*, music player, soft rhythmic music selections, paper, pens, pencils, crayons, colored markers or pencils

Greet everyone and ask if there are any questions before getting started. Once questions have been addressed, ask each person to share their homework by reading aloud or telling their story of life after the trauma. Notice anyone who is able to connect with feelings as they tell their story of life after the trauma and allow ample time for the expression and sharing of those feelings, as members are able to share. If they are unable to find language to share the feelings, provide paper and crayons or markers and suggest they draw out those feelings for themselves. Ask them to focus on where the feelings are occurring in their bodies. Encourage and reinforce the decision to share the experience with others. Once everyone has had opportunity to share and discuss the homework, begin this lesson.

The Pot of Gold at the End of the Rainbow (modified from an activity first presented by Karen Hutchison, in Kaduson and Schaefer, 2003).

The group leader begins by playing some calm, soothing, relaxing music. Lead the group members in the deep breathing exercise from previous meetings. Have members close their eyes as they practice their deep breathing. Once the group members have taken several long, slow, deep breaths as they listen to the soothing music, give these instructions: "Imagine you are sitting looking out your window. Outside the window is the aftermath of your traumatic experience. What do you see? Draw for me whatever you see when you are looking out your window." Keep the music playing throughout the drawing activity. Once everyone is finished with their drawing, ask if anyone would like to share what they have drawn. Some members may choose not to share, which is perfectly fine. Others may express some emotions as they share. Encourage their expression of feelings with your calm and soothing, slow-paced responses. Pay attention to members who may be shutting down or avoiding their feelings and those who may be overwhelmed by their feelings. Remember to stop the activity to assist anyone who has difficulty with emotional regulation, utilizing mindfulness, breathing, and the other strategies discussed in the model's instructions. Encourage them to continue breathing deeply and focusing on where in their bodies their feelings are expressed.

When this part of the activity is over, continue with these instructions: "Now, close your eyes again, and imagine that it is gently raining outside your window. (If you have some music that includes the sounds of rain or is reminiscent of rain, you can play that music during this part of the activity). Watch how the rain washes and cleanses everything. See how the land takes in the water and how the plants get greener and begin growing because of the refreshing rain. Now look up into the sky and watch as the clouds part, and the sun comes out from behind the clouds. Look! A rainbow is forming, coming down out of the sky until it touches the ground. Look at all the beautiful colors of the rainbow. Now open your eyes and draw the scene that you saw outside your window."

As the group members are drawing, continue to play the soothing music. Once the drawings are completed, the group leader can comment on the drawings, how beautiful the rainbows are, etc. The leader then talks about how legend says that every rainbow has a pot of gold at the end of it. Tell the group members the gold is like a special treasure that signals the end of the storm. Ask them what they believe will be in their pot of gold at the end of their rainbow. Allow each person to share, if they choose to do so. End the activity by having them draw their individual treasure that they imagine is in their pot of gold. Encourage them to take their drawings home with them, reinforcing that the pot of gold is their special treasure that means the storm has ended.

Always encourage and remind members to notice what is going on within their bodies at all times. Explain to them how paying attention to what is going on within them helps to connect them to their feelings and reconnect their memories to their bodies, which aids in healing.

Once the exercise is completed and everyone has had the opportunity to share, ask the group to review the previous portions of the story by asking, "Who can share with me what has happened in the story so far?" After a brief review, begin this exercise.

I Get to Write my Own Story

Read Part IV (pages 23-24) of Caonaciba's story and reflect on what defined his life after the trauma.

Ask and discuss the following questions:

What happened in this last part of Caonaciba's story?

What was his life like in the last part?

What happened to his beliefs?

What happened to his values?

What was his reality now?

Then, shift to a discussion of the participants' lives. Ask the following questions:

How are you like Caonaciba?

Reflect on defining your life from now on.

What direction do you want to take in your life?

What are you going to do?

How do you feel?

Is the trauma going to define the rest of your life or are you going to define the rest of your life?

What happens now to your beliefs?

What happens now to your values?

What is your reality going to be?

Have each person share their reflections and have the group discuss them. Be attentive, kind, and supportive and encourage all the group members to listen attentively and support the others as they share. Reinforce appropriate behavior and thank each person as they share by letting them know that you understand how hard it can be to talk about difficult personal things.

Once the discussion is completed, share the following homework exercise for them to complete before the next meeting.

Homework: Explain how some people allow a traumatic event to determine how their lives will be from then on, and how some people choose for themselves how their lives will be in spite of the trauma. Remind them how Caonaciba learned to choose his own course for his life. Have each person write or draw or tell how they will define their lives from now on. Tell them they will share their homework for the next lesson. Encourage them to do this assignment with their loved ones (family members, friends, or support system).

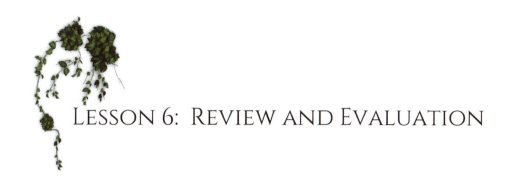

Lesson 6: Review and Evaluation

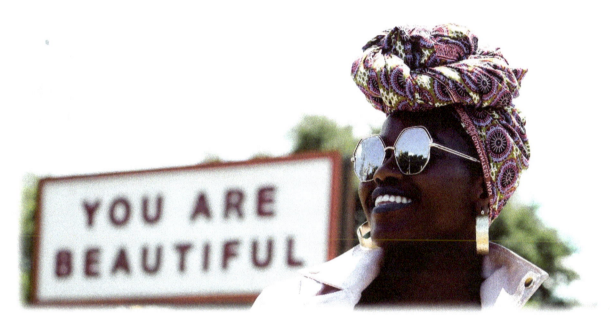

You have a true identity — a true "name" that defines you, reflecting your inner beauty and everything that makes you valuable and unique

Supplies needed: paper, pens, pencils, crayons, colored markers or pencils, magazines, scissors, glue sticks, music player, soothing and rhythmic music selections

Greet everyone and ask if there are any questions before getting started. Once questions have been addressed, ask each person to share their homework by reading aloud or telling how they will define their lives from now on. Notice anyone who is able to connect with feelings as they tell their story of how they will define their lives from now on and allow ample time for the expression and sharing of those feelings, as members are able to share. If they are unable to find language to share the feelings, provide paper and crayons or markers and suggest they draw out those feelings for themselves. Ask them to focus on where the feelings are occurring in their bodies. For those who worked on the homework with loved ones, reinforce the decision to share the experience with others. Once everyone has had opportunity to share and discuss the homework, begin this lesson.

The Buried Treasure

Begin by reminding members how Caonaciba's namesake was the Gold Stone, which defined him before the trauma, but after the trauma he lost connection with his true self and his true name. Through the help of his guides, Caonaciba was able to reconnect with his true self and reclaim his true name. Then, share the following: "Like Caonaciba, you have a true identity; a true "name" that defines you. Just like a beautiful gold stone, when it is out in the sunlight, uniquely captures and reflects light and colors, your identity reflects your inner beauty and everything that makes you valuable, unique, and one-of-a-kind. Sometimes, though, gold stones get covered up by dirt that is piled up on them over time. 'Dirt' represents traumatic circumstances that happen to us and beliefs we come to have about ourselves as a result of those hurts from our past. The dirt might hide the gold stone, and the dirt might keep the gold from shining with its unique color and light, but it does not change the gold, because the gold is much stronger than the dirt. In order for your gold to once again shine, you brush the dirt off of it and bring it back out into the light. And that is what we are going to do in this activity."

Instruct each member to write one word in the center of a piece of paper that they believe in the deepest part of their hearts is true of them. Encourage group members to choose a word that reflects an inner truth of their nature rather than something external. Other than that instruction, their word can be anything they choose. Some examples they might choose include words such as "caring" or "survivor" or "sensitive" or "strong-willed" or "determined."

Have each member share their unique word and discuss it briefly. Then, for each word shared, ask the group to call out words that they know are true of people who are described by that word. For example, if someone chooses the word, "sensitive," the group might call out, "loving, quiet, calm, giving, easily hurt, compassionate, warm."

Have the member write all the words called out on their paper in a circle around their central word. Complete this exercise for each member. Once everyone has created a composite of all the descriptors shared for them, inform the members that this paper is their "treasure;" that it is unique and one-of-a-kind; and, most importantly, it is not defined by the trauma. Allow members to discuss how it feels to see themselves in this way, as described by those words. Have the members take their "treasure" page home to keep, to remind them who they are.

Once everyone has had ample opportunity to share, continue to the following exercise.

Picturing the treasure: As time allows, and if materials are available, place several magazines of different kinds around for each member, as well as scissors and glue. Ask members to cut out pictures to create a collage that represents their "treasure" (who they truly are), using pictures they cut out from the magazines. Play soft, soothing music in the background as the group members create their collages. Allow members to share their collages and discuss them with each other. If these resources are not available, transition to the next exercise.

Drawings

Re-do two of the drawings from the first meeting. Play soft, soothing, rhythmic music as they complete the drawings, and remind members to breathe deeply and slowly and pay attention to their breathing as they draw. Compare these drawings rto the first set of drawings to give members an idea of the progress they have made.

This is Me: I am… This drawing shows you what you think about yourself. It is your self-portrait.

My Space. This drawing shows how you see your world, your position in it, and your reaction to it. Do you believe you have a space in your world? What are your relationships with significant others? Where do your fears, wishes, anger, depression, and personal strengths and weakness fit in? How do you tolerate your world in the present? Do you feel isolated and withdrawn or included and part of the world around you?

Discuss the similarities and differences in each of these drawings with those drawings made earlier. Allow members to process their views on how they have grown and changed through their experiences. In any ways the members see positive growth and changes, reinforce those changes are constant and continued growth and changes are possible, remembering that trauma survivors often feel "frozen" or "stuck" in the trauma.

After each drawing, ask who wants to share and discuss the drawings and what they mean.

Wrap up by asking if there are any other questions or comments. Thank everyone for participating in the group. Remind them they now have the ability to decide how their life moves forward. Unfortunately, bad things happen in life, but they are not defined by those events. Explain how they are now equipped to deal with trauma, difficult times, and adversity as it happens by applying the things they have learned and experienced. Allow group members to develop a ritual or ceremony to celebrate completion of the group. Leave them with this encouragement: Remember these lessons and choose to write a meaningful story.

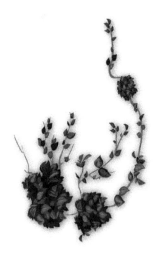

Choose to write

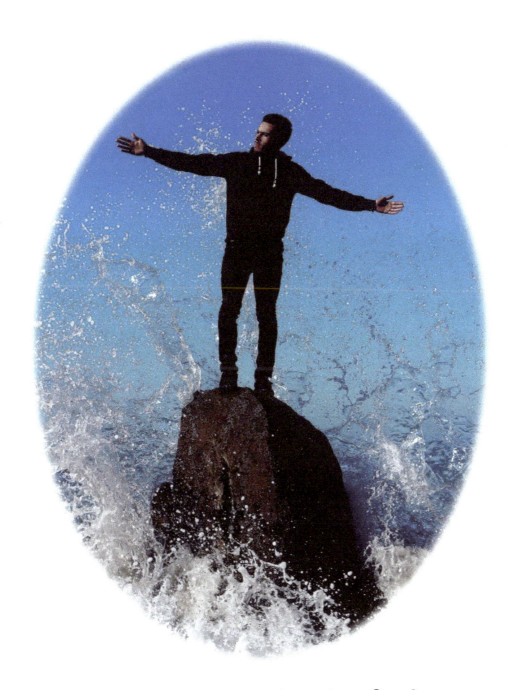

a meaningful story

BIBLIOGRAPHY

American Psychiatric Association. (1994). *Diagnostic and Statistical Manual of Mental Disorders,* 4th ed. Washington, D.C.: American Psychiatric Association.

Angus, L. E., & McLeod, J. (2004). *The handbook of narrative and psychotherapy: Practice, theory, and research.* Thousand Oaks, CA: Sage Publications, Inc.

Baker, G.R., and M. Salston. (1993). *Management of intrusion and arousal symptoms in PTSD.* San Diego: Association for Traumatic Stress Specialists (International Association for Trauma Counselors).

Beaudoin, M. N. (2005). *Agency and choice in the face of trauma: A narrative therapy map.* Journal of Systemic Therapies, *24*(4), 32-50. doi: 10.1521/jsyt.2005.24.4.32

Booker, J., Gracie, M., Hudak, L., Jovanovis, T. Rothbaum, B., Ressler, K., Fivush, R., & Stevens, J. (2018). *Narratives in the immediate aftermath of traumatic injury: Markers of ongoing depressive and posttraumatic stress disorder symptoms.* Journal of Traumatic Stress, Vol. 31(2).

Bowlby, J. (1980). *Attachment and loss.* New York, NY: Basic Books.

Briere, J. N., & Scott, C. (2015). *Principles of trauma therapy: A guide to symptoms, evaluation, and treatment* (2nd ed.). Los Angeles, CA: Sage.

Carless, D. & Douglas, K. (2016). *Narrating embodied experience: Sharing stories of trauma and recovery.* Sport, Education, and Society, Vol. 21(1).

Cattanach, A. (2008). Working creatively with children and their families after trauma: The storied life. In C. A. Malchiodi (Ed.), *Creative interventions with traumatized children.* (pp. 211-224). New York, NY: Guilford Press.

Colson, Denise A. (2004). *Stop Treating Symptoms and Start Resolving Trauma: Inside-Out Healing for Survivors of All Types.* Author House, Bloomington, IN

Crawford, Allison (2010). *If "the body keeps the score": Mapping the dissociated body in trauma narrative, intervention, and theory.* University of Toronto Quarterly Vol 79, 2.

Crossley, M. L. (2000). *Introducing narrative psychology: Self, trauma and the construction of meaning.* Maidenhead, BRK England: Open University Press.

Davidson, J. R. T., Book, S. W., Colket, J. T., Tupler, L. A., Roth, S., David, D., Hertzberg, M., Mellman, T., Beckham, J. C., Smith, R., Davison, R. M., Katz, R., & Feldman, M. (1997). *Assessment of a new self-rating scale for post-traumatic stress disorder.* Psychological Medicine, 27, 153-160.

Davidson, J. R., Tharwani, H. M., Connor, K. M. (2002). *Davidson Trauma Scale (DTS): Normative scores in the general population and effect sizes in placebo-controlled SSRI trials.* Depression and Anxiety, 15, 75-78.

Dingfelder, S. F. (2011). *Our stories, ourselves.* American Psychological Association: Monitor Staff, 42.

Donovan, T. (2018). *Reclaiming lives from sexual violence.* International Journal of Narrative Therapy & Community Work, Issue 1.

Foa, E.B., & Rothbaum, B. O. (1998). *Treating the trauma of rape: Cognitive-behavioral therapy for PTSD.* New York: Guilford.

Frechette, C. (2017). *Two Biblical motifs of divine violence as resources for meaning-making in engaging self-blame and rage after traumatization.* Pastoral Psychology, Vol. 66 Issue 2.

Gerge, A. & Pedersen, I. (2017). *Analyzing pictorial artifacts from psychotherapy and art therapy when overcoming stress and trauma.* The Arts in Psychotherapy, Vol 54, 56-68.

Hall, S., Broder, K., LaBar, K., Berntsen, D., & Rubin, D. (2018). *Neural responses to emotional involuntary memories in posttraumatic stress disorder: Differences in timing and activity.* Neuroimage: Clinical, Volume 19, 793-804.

Harrington, S., Morrison, O., & Pascal-Leone, A. (2018). *Emotional processing in an expressive writing task on trauma.* Complimentary Therapies in Clinical Practice, Volume 32, 116-122.

Hass-Cohen, N., Bokoch, R., Findlay, J., & Witting, A. (2017). *A four drawing art therapy trauma and resiliency protocol study.* The Arts in Psychotherapy.

Herman, Judith L. (1997). *Trauma & recovery.* New York, NY: Basic Books.

Hutto, D., Brancazio, N., & Aubourg, J. (2017). *Narrative practices in medicine and therapy: Philosophical reflections.* Pennsylvania State University Press, Vol 51 Issue 3.

Iacona, J. & Johnson, S. (2018). *Neurobiology of trauma and mindfulness for children.* Journal of Trauma Nursing, 25(3).

Johnson, J. (2018). *Awakening to hope through narrative practices.* International Journal of Narrative Therapy & Community Work, Issue 1.

Kaduson, H. and Schaefer, C. eds. (2003). *101 Favorite Play Therapy Techniques Volume III.* Northvale, NJ: Jason Aronson Inc.

Kalmanowitz, D. & Ho, R. (2017). *Art therapy and mindfulness with survivors of political violence: A qualitative study.* Psychological Trauma: Theory, Research, Practice, and Policy, Vol 9.

Kaminer, D. (2006). *Healing processes in trauma narratives: A review.* South African Journal of Psychology, 36(3), 481-499.

Kamya, H. (2012). The cultural universality of narrative techniques in the creation of meaning. In R. A. McMackin, E. Newman, J. M. Fogler & T. M. Keane (Eds.), *Trauma therapy in context: The science and craft of evidence-based practice.* (pp. 231-245). Washington, DC: American Psychological Association.

Lane, W. David, Myers, Keith J., and Lane, Donna E. (2017). *Brief narrative trauma treatment with survivors of natural disaster.* Kentucky Journal of Professional Counseling, Issue 1, Volume II.

Lane, W. David, Myers, Keith J., Hill, Maurice C., and Lane, Donna E. (2015). *Utilizing narrative methodology in trauma treatment with Haitian earthquake survivors.* Journal of Loss and Trauma, Volume 21, Issue 6.

Langer, L. L. (1991). *Holocaust Testimonies: The Ruins of Memory.* New Haven: Yale University Press.

Leahy, R. L. (2009). *Those damn unwanted thoughts.* Psychology Today.

Madigan, S. (2010). *Narrative Therapy (Theories of Psychotherapy).* Washington D.C.: American Psychological Association.

Marshall, E. & Frazier, P. (2018). *Understanding posttrauma reactions within an attachment theory framework.* Current Opinion in Psychology.

Matos, M., Santos, A., Gonçalves, M., & Martins, C. (2009). *Innovative moments and change in narrative therapy*. Psychotherapy Research, 19(1), 68-80.

McKinnon, A., Brewer, N., Maiser-Stedman, R., & Nixon, R. (2017). *Trauma memory characteristics and the development of acute stress disorder and post-traumatic stress disorder in youth*. Journal of Behavior Therapy and Experimental Psychiatry, Volume 54, 112-119.

Meichenbaum, D. (1994). *A Clinical Handbook/Practical Therapist Manual: For Assessing and Treating Adults with Post-Traumatic Stress Disorder.* Waterloo, Ont.: Institute Press.

Meichenbaum, D. (2000). *Treating patients with PTSD: A constructive narrative approach*. Clinical Quarterly 9(4):55, 58-59.

Meichenbaum, D. (2017). A constructive narrative perspective on trauma and resilience: The role of cognitive and affective processes. In Gold, S., Ed., *APA Handbook of Trauma Psychology: Foundations in Knowledge.* Washington D.C.: American Psychological Association.

Menard, R., Robinson, K., Lane, D. E., and Lane, W. D. (2018). *Group approach to narrative therapy: A review of the literature.* Journal of Counseling Research and Practice, Volume 3, Number 1.

O'Connor, M., & Elklit, A. (2008). *Attachment styles, traumatic events, and PTSD: A cross-sectional investigation of adult attachment and trauma.* Attachment & Human Development, 10(1), 59-71.

Olafson, E., Boat, B., Putnam, K., Thieken, L. Marrow, M. & Putnam, F. (2018). *Implementing trauma and grief component therapy for adolescents and think trauma for traumatized youth in secure juvenile justice settings.* Journal of Interpersonal Violence, Vol 33 Issue 16.

Oncu, E., & Wise, A. (2010). *The effects of the 1999 Turkish earthquake on young children: Analyzing traumatized children's completion of short stories.* Child Development, 81(4), 1161-1175.

Pack, Margaret (2008). *Back from the edge of the world: Re-authoring a story of practice with stress and trauma using Gestalt and Narrative approaches.* Journal of Systemic Therapies, Vol. 27, 3.

Pennebaker, J.W. (1997). *Opening Up: The Healing Power of Expressing Emotions.* New York: Guilford Press.

Perdomo, C. (2018). *Undocumented and deportable: Re-authoring trauma within the context of immigration in a narrative-informed single session.* Journal of Systemic Therapies, Vol 36 Issue 4.

Plokar, A., Bisaillon, C., & Terradas, M. (2018). *Development of the child dissociation assessment system using a narrative story stem task: A preliminary study.* European Journal of Trauma and Dissociation, 2(1).

Porter, E. (2016). *Gendered narratives: Stories and silences in transitional justice.* Human Rights Review, Vol. 17 Issue 1.

Price, M., Spinnazola, J., Musicaro, R., Turner, J., Suvak, M., Emerson, D., & Van der Kolk, B. (2017). *Effectiveness of extended yoga treatment for women with chronic posttraumatic stress disorder.* Journal of Alternative & Complimentary Medicine, 23(4).

Rhodes, A., Spinnazola, J., & Van der Kolk, B. (2016). *Yoga for adult women with chronic PTSD: A long-term follow-up study.* Journal of Alternative & Complimentary Medicine, 22(3).

Rosenbloom, D., and M.B. Williams. (1999). *Life After Trauma: A Workbook for Healing.* New York: Guilford Press.

Rothschild, B. (2000). *The Body Remembers*: *The Psychophysiology of Trauma and Trauma Treatment.* New York: W.W. Norton.

Schauer, M., Neuner, F., & Elbert, T. (2011). *Narrative exposure therapy: A short-term treatment for traumatic stress disorders (2nd ed.).* Cambridge, MA: Hogrefe Publishing.

Scheib, K. (2016). *Pastoral Care: Telling the Stories of Our Lives.* Nashville: Abingdon Press.

Shaw, A., Joseph, S., & Linley, P. A. (2005). *Religion, spirituality, and post-traumatic growth: A systematic review.* Mental Health, Religion & Culture, 8(1), 1-11.

Stewart, A. E., & Neimeyer, R. A. (2007). Emplotting the traumatic self: Narrative revision and the construction of coherence. In S. Krippner, M. Bova & L. Gray (Eds.), *Healing stories: The use of narrative in counseling and psychotherapy.* (pp. 41-62). San Juan Puerto Rico: Puente Publications.

Tedeschi, R. G., & Calhoun, L. G. (2004). *Post-traumatic growth: Conceptual foundations and empirical evidence.* Psychological Inquiry, 15(1), 1-18.

Tedeschi, R. G., C. L. Park, and L. G. Calhoun, eds. (1998). *Post Traumatic Growth: Positive Changes in the Aftermath of Crisis.* Mahweh, NJ.: Lawrence Erlbaum Associates, Inc., Publishers.

Thomason, M. & Marusak, H. (2017). *Toward understanding the impact of trauma on early brain development.* Neurosciences, Volume 342, 55-67.

Thomson, P. & Jaque, S. (2017). *Adverse childhood experiences (ACE) and adult attachment interview (AAI) in a non-clinical population.* Child Abuse and Neglect, 70, 255-263.

Ursano, R. J., Grieger, T. A., & McCarroll, J. E. (2007). Prevention of post-traumatic stress consultation, training, and early treatment. In Van der Kolk, B. A., McFarlane, A. C., & Weisath, L. (Eds.), *Traumatic Stress: The effects of overwhelming experience on mind, body, and society.* New York, NY: The Guilford Press.

Van der Kolk, B. A. (2014). *The Body Keeps the Score: Brain, Mind, and Body in the healing of trauma.* New York, NY: Viking.

Van der Kolk, B. A. (1999). The body keeps the score: Memory and the evolving psychobiology of post-traumatic stress. In M. J. Horowitz (Ed.), *Essential papers on post-traumatic stress disorder.* (pp. 301-326). New York, NY: New York University Press.

Van der Kolk, B.A. (1996). *Traumatic Stress: The effects of overwhelming experience on mind, body and society.* New York: Guilford Press.

Van der Velden, P. G., Wong, A., Boshuizen, H. C., & Grievink, L. (2013). *Persistent mental health disturbances during the 10 years after a disaster: Four-wave longitudinal comparative study.* Psychiatry and Clinical Neurosciences, 67(2), 110-118.

White, M. (2007). *Maps of Narrative Practice.* New York, NY: W.W. Norton & Company, Inc.

White, M., & Epston, D. (1990). *Narrative Means to Therapeutic Ends.* New York, NY: W.W. Norton & Company, Inc.

Zang, Y., Hunt, N., & Cox, T. (2013). *A randomised controlled pilot study: The effectiveness of narrative exposure therapy with adult survivors of the Sichuan earthquake.* BMC Psychiatry, 13.

Zerrudo, M. (2016). *Theater of disaster, folk stories as vehicles for healing and survival.* Teaching Artist Journal, 14(3).

About the Authors

W. David Lane

W. David Lane, Ph.D., Professor, Department of Counseling, Penfield College of Mercer University, is the founder of the Counseling Program and Ph.D. program at Mercer University in Atlanta. He earned the Ph.D. in Counseling from Georgia State University in 1992, and has been a counselor, counselor educator, and supervisor since 1978. David is a Licensed Professional Counselor, a Licensed Marriage and Family Therapist, a Nationally Board Certified Counselor, a Certified Professional Counselor Supervisor, and a Clinical Member of the American Association for Marriage and Family Therapists. He has been at Mercer University since 1995. He was awarded the Dr. Linda Painter Service Award and the Dr. John C. Burns Lifetime Achievement Award for Counseling in 2018.

He has published numerous articles, book chapters, and manuscript reviews in the field of Counseling and Marriage and Family Therapy. He is the co-author of *Ready to Learn: Teaching Children How to Succeed in School*, a national award-winning program for pre-school and early childhood classrooms; *Please Share the Door, I'm Freezing: Creating Oneness in Marriage*, a Christian marriage workbook co-authored with his wife, Donna; and, *Strength in Adversity*, also co-authored with Donna. He is co-author of *Strength in Our Story*, a study of the Biblical Joseph story based on *Trauma Narrative Treatment*. He and Donna also co-authored *Gold Stone*, the story used as the basis for this model. He is a regular presenter at local, regional, national, and international workshops in the field of counseling.

After the earthquake in Haiti in 2010, David worked extensively for over a year in Haiti leading teams of professionals to train pastors, teachers, and mental health providers in trauma assessment and care. In the wake of the Newtown, CT, Sandy Hook School shootings in 2012, David led two teams to train pastors and community workers to assist with the trauma.

Donna E. Lane

Dr. Donna Lane is an author, Adjunct Professor of Counseling at Mercer University, and a Christian Counselor in private practice since 1993. She is founder of the Cody Lane Foundation, which provides individual and small group discipleship and Christian education. She has presented at local, regional, national, and international conferences and workshops on such topics as trauma, grief and loss, marriage counseling, toxic religion, early childhood education, parenting, narrative therapy, counselor education, clergy in crisis, and soul care. She participated in training workshops for pastors and community workers in Newtown, CT, following the shootings at Sandy Hook.

She co-authored the award-winning *Ready to Learn* series, which teaches preschoolers and elementary students needed learning skills. With her husband, David, she co-authored the Christian marriage workbook, *Please Share the Door, I'm Freezing: Creating Oneness in Marriage*, *Strength in Adversity*, a Biblical study on handling adversity through faith, and *Gold Stone*, the story used as the basis for this curriculum. With her son, Hayden Lane, she co-authored the book, *Restored Christianity*, which is currently in its second edition. She is the author of *The Interview*, a Christian fictional allegory of trauma as representative of evil, and *Wilderness Meditations,* a 40-day devotional for Lent. She is also co-author of *Strength in Our Story,* a study of the Biblical Joseph story based on *Trauma Narrative Treatment.*

Donna and David have been married since 1979, and have three wonderful children; Hayden, Lindsey, and Cody, who passed away in 2007 after a battle with a degenerative neurological disorder. Their personal journey through grief and loss has informed much of their writing on trauma and grief.

The Artists
(in order of presentation)

Lars Nissen (cover art)
Aziz Acharki
Carolina Heza
Pawel Szvmans
Caleb Jones
Alex Iby
Bekah Russom
Luis Galvez
David Lane
Anonymous
Gavin Hang
William Farlow
Jacek Dylag
Ieva Vizule
Darius Bashar
Anonymous
Eric Brolin
Rawpixel
Mantas Hesthaven
Hugues deBuyer Mimeure
Geralt
Marie Paddock
Sydney Sims
Jared Erondu
Hannah Grace
Aziz Acharki

Other Titles by These Authors

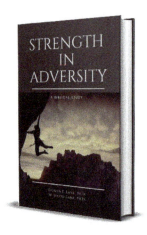
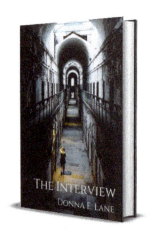
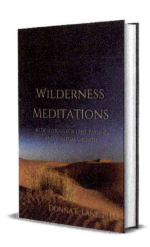
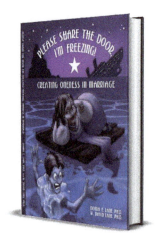
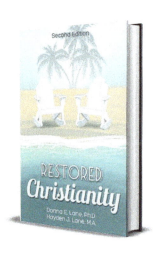
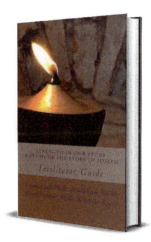

CPSIA information can be obtained
at www.ICGtesting.com
Printed in the USA
LVHW071604300322
714781LV00009B/360